Your Operation

Hernias

Other titles published in this series

Breast lumps
Hysterectomy & alternative operations
Varicose veins (published in 1993 by Claremont Press)

Your Operation

Hernias

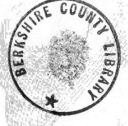

Jane Smith *BSc (Hons)*
Medical Editor and Writer, Bristol

&

David J. Leaper *MD, ChM, FRCS*
Consultant and Senior Lecturer in Surgery,
University of Bristol, Southmead Hospital, Bristol

ILLUSTRATIONS BY ALEXANDER JAMES

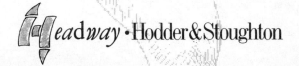

British Library Cataloguing in Publication Data
Leaper, David J.
  Hernias. – (Your Operation Series)
  I. Title   II. Smith, Jane III. Series
  617.559

ISBN 0 340 620471

First published 1994
Impression number   10 9 8 7 6 5 4 3 2 1
Year   1998 1997 1996 1995 1994

Typeset by Wearset, Boldon, Tyne and Wear.
Printed in Great Britain for Hodder & Stoughton Educational, a division of
Hodder Headline Plc, 338 Euston Road, London NW1 3BH by
Cox & Wyman Limited, Reading

Contents

General preface
to the series

Two people having the same operation can have quite different experiences, but one feeling that is common to many is that things might have been easier if they had had a better idea of what to expect. Some people are reluctant to ask questions, and many forget what they are told, sometimes because they are anxious, and sometimes because they do not really understand the explanations they are given.

The emphasis in most medical centres in Britain today is more on patient involvement than at any time in the past. It is now generally accepted that it is important for people to understand what their treatment entails, both in terms of reducing their stress and thus aiding their recovery, and of making their care more straightforward for the medical staff involved.

The books in this series have been written with the aim of giving people comprehensive information about each of the medical conditions covered, about the treatment they are likely to be offered, and about what may happen during their post-operative recovery period. Armed with this knowledge, you should have the confidence to question, and to take part in the decisions made.

Going in to hospital for the first time can be a daunting experience, and therefore the books describe the procedures involved, and identify and explain the roles of the hospital staff with whom you are likely to come into contact.

Anaesthesia is explained in general terms, and the options available for a particular operation are described in each book.

There may be complications following any operation – usually minor but none the less worrying for the person involved – and the common ones are described and explained. Now that less time is spent in hospital following most non-emergency operations, knowing what to expect in the days following surgery, and what to do if a complication does arise, is more important than ever before.

Where relevant, the books include a section of exercises and advice to help you to get back to normal and to deal with the everyday activities which can be difficult or painful in the first few days after an operation.

Doctors and nurses, like members of any profession, use a jargon, and they often forget that many of the terms that are familiar to them are not part of everyday language for most of us. Care has been taken to make the books easily understandable by everyone, and each book has a list of simple explanations of the medical terms you may come across.

Most doctors and nurses are more than willing to explain and to discuss problems with patients, but they often assume that if you do not ask questions, you either do not want to know or you know already. Questions and answers are given in every book to help you to draw up your own list to take with you when you see your GP or consultant.

Each book also has a section of case histories of people who have actually experienced the particular operation themselves. These are included to give you an idea of the problems which can arise, problems which may sometimes seem relatively trivial to others but which can be distressing to those directly concerned.

Although the majority of people are satisfied with the medical care they receive, things can go wrong. If you do feel you need to make a complaint about something that happened, or did not happen, during your treatment, each book has a section which deals in detail with how to go about this.

It was the intention in writing these books to help to take some of the worry out of having an operation. It is not knowing what to expect, and the feeling of being involved in some process over which we have no control, and which we do not fully understand, that makes us anxious. The books in the series *Your Operation* should help to remove some of that anxiety and make you feel less like a car being serviced, and more like part of the team of people who are working together to cure your medical problem and put you back on the road to health.

You may not know *all* there is to know about a particular condition when you have read the book related to it, but you will know more than enough to prepare yourself for your operation. You may decide you do not want to go ahead with surgery. Although this is not the authors' intention, they will be happy that you have been given enough information to feel confident to make your own decision, and to take an active part in your own care. After all, it is *your* operation.

Jane Smith
Bristol, 1994

Preface

The majority of the hernia operations carried out in Britain each year – some 100 000 in all – are to repair hernias in the groin. Hernias are common in both men and women, and can occur in children, even in babies. Although they can develop in many parts of the body, they are most common in the abdomen, and it is these abdominal hernias which are dealt with in detail in this book.

Hiatus hernias, which are diaphragmatic rather than abdominal, are described briefly, with some suggestions of possible ways of relieving their symptoms. They present rather different problems from the abdominal hernias themselves. Surgical treatment is rarely required for hiatus hernias but, when it is necessary, it is a more complex, major procedure, and therefore is not described here.

The surgical repair of abdominal hernias is usually carried out to relieve troublesome symptoms, and to prevent complications arising in the future, but in some cases surgery is required as an emergency. However, an operation is not always necessary, and some people live with their hernias for many years.

Going in to hospital can be a daunting prospect, particularly for those who have never had an operation before; knowing what to expect can help to relieve some of the anxiety. This book gives clear descriptions of the different types of hernias and how they develop, and describes in simple language all aspects of their treatment.

You are likely to be in hospital for only one or two days following a straightforward hernia operation, and in some cases no overnight stay will be involved. Although many people are glad to return home so quickly, the prospect of having to take responsibility for their own recovery may be worrying. Knowing what is likely to happen, what can go wrong, and when to seek medical advice, is reassuring – both for those undergoing treatment and for those who will help to care for them after their operation.

When learning about something with which we are unfamiliar, we do not always absorb new facts the first time we come across them. The occasional repetition in this book is therefore intentional, with this in mind.

We hope the book answers the questions you may have about your hernia and its treatment and that, having read it, you will feel more confident about your forthcoming stay in hospital.

Jane Smith
David J. Leaper
Bristol, 1994

Acknowledgements

This book could not have been written without the help of the many people who gave so generously of their time and knowledge.

We would like to thank Dr Alasdair Dow, Senior Registrar in Anaesthetics at the Royal Devon and Exeter Hospital, for the chapter on anaesthesia; and Mr Scott Watkin, formerly Staff Grade Surgeon at Southmead Hospital, Bristol, for his chapter on laparoscopic hernia repair.

We are particularly grateful to Dr Ian Donaldson, GP; to Ward Sister Judy Vickery; to Superintendent Physiotherapist Mrs Sandra Farmer; to Mrs Rose West and all the staff at The BUPA Hospital Bristol; and to Mr John Loosley of the Bristol & District Community Health Council.

Finally, we would like to thank the men and women who gave up their time to talk to us and whose experiences we have described in the section of case histories.

CHAPTER ONE

Introduction

A hernia is a swelling caused by an organ, or part of an organ, pushing through an opening in a muscle wall and thus protruding out of the body cavity in which it is normally found. Hernias are most common in the abdomen, and there are several different types which can develop in men, women and children at any age. Before being able to understand how these arise, it is useful to have an idea of the structure of the parts of the body in which they usually occur.

THE HUMAN BODY

The cavities of the human body contain organs, as well as blood vessels, nerves and glands. The abdomen, or **abdominal cavity**, is the largest, and most of its organs are involved with digestion or the breakdown and excretion of waste products. These include the liver, spleen, kidneys, stomach, small bowel and colon. The abdomen is separated from the chest, or **thoracic cavity**, by a thin sheet of muscle called the **diaphragm**. The organs in the chest are the lungs, heart, windpipe and gullet. The lower abdomen is continuous with the pelvis, or **pelvic cavity**, which contains the bladder, the rectum, and some reproductive organs. The floor of the pelvis is formed by the muscles of the pelvic diaphragm.

The abdominal cavity and its organs are lined by a thin membrane called the **peritoneum**. The peritoneum allows the organs to move within the abdomen without sticking to each other or to the abdominal wall.

Although most hernias are abdominal, they can occur in other parts of the body, such as the skull or thoracic cavity. Only the abdominal hernias will be dealt with in detail in this book, although hiatus hernias – commonly occurring diaphragmatic hernias – are described briefly in Chapter 11.

WHAT ARE HERNIAS?

A hernia consists of a bag or sac of peritoneum which may contain some of the contents of the abdominal cavity, such as a loop of the small bowel. The peritoneal sac may narrow into a 'neck' as it passes through a gap in the muscles of the abdominal wall; it then bulges out to form the hernial sac.

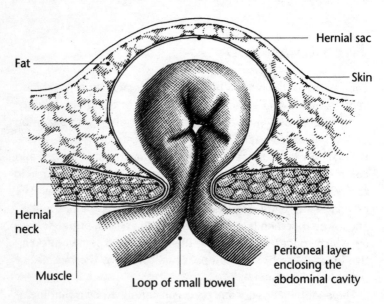

A hernia. A defect in the abdominal wall has allowed a loop of bowel to protrude into a hernial sac.

The muscles in the walls of the abdomen are usually firm and hold the organs in place. If these muscles become slack, due to overstraining or because of some weakness present from birth, a hernia may force its way through or between them.

Hernias can form at any naturally occurring weak spot, such as the umbilicus, or at a scar. Numerous structures, including nerves, blood vessels and tendons, run through the body in canals, and weak spots can also occur where these canals enter and leave the body cavities.

Causes of hernias

Hernias usually occur when the peritoneal sac pushes through an *existing* weakness in the abdominal muscle wall. If strenuous activity causes the muscles of the wall to split suddenly, a hernia may form immediately, although many develop gradually as the tissues weaken with age.

Hernias can occasionally be the result of an injury, caused, for example, by a knife or gunshot wound or a car crash. The muscle wall can also be weakened by surgery, such as an appendix operation, particularly if there has been an infection. More often, the weakness in the muscle wall is congenital – that is, it will have been present since birth. Although hernias are fairly common in babies and small children, most appear later in life, the weakness only becoming apparent as the years go by.

Some people are predisposed to develop hernias as a result of being overweight; repeated pregnancies also cause weakening of the muscle walls. In the front of the abdomen, on either side of the midline, there is a vertical, strap-like column of muscle called the rectus muscle. A potential weakness exists between the two columns, and when a gap opens up, the condition is known as **divarication of the recti**. The abdominal contents can herniate through this gap. However, as the gap is wide, complications are unlikely, and an operation to correct the condition is not usually necessary.

COMPLICATIONS OF HERNIAS

Strangulation

If the contents of the hernial sac cannot easily be pushed back into the abdomen, their blood supply may become cut off. The affected part may then become gangrenous and die due to lack of oxygen. The hernia becomes enlarged, becoming tense and painful, and the skin over it will redden. If this happens, an urgent operation will be necessary. The hernia will change from a soft swelling to a hard, painful lump. **Seek urgent medical attention immediately if this occurs.**

Richter's hernias develop when only part of the circumference of the bowel, rather than an entire section, is strangulated within the sac. Some of the bowel's contents are therefore still able to pass through it. This may lead to confusion if obstruction of the bowel is suspected and the patient is vomiting but also has diarrhoea. Richter's hernias are usually femoral (see p.9).

Obstruction

If a hernia has bulged through a *small* gap in the muscle wall, the passage of food through the intestine may be blocked, although the blood supply to the trapped gut will not be affected. Obstruction will lead to loss of appetite and a swollen belly. Wind and faeces may no longer be passed through the anus, and belching increases, as does discomfort. Nausea gives way to vomiting, first of the last food eaten, then of bile and finally, if the condition remains untreated, of waste matter from the bowel. This is often accompanied by spasms of abdominal pain. Again, **urgent surgery is required if obstruction occurs**.

TYPES OF HERNIA

Each of the several different types of hernia is named after the part of the body in which it occurs. A hernia of some sort is present in approximately 1 in every 100 people.

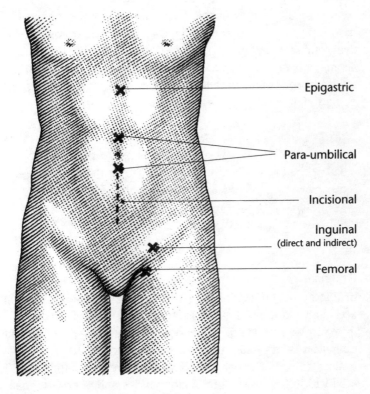

Epigastric

Para-umbilical

Incisional

Inguinal
(direct and indirect)

Femoral

Common hernia sites. Abdominal hernias can occur at any of the sites indicated in this diagram. The broken line shows the area in which incisional hernias can develop.

Umbilical hernias

These are the most common congenital hernias. The abdominal muscle wall of a newborn baby may not develop fully, and babies are sometimes born with a small bulge around the navel. Because the hole in the abdominal muscle wall is large, often bigger than a golf ball, there is little danger of the gut becoming stuck and causing complications. However, strangulation of the bowel is a slight risk in large umbilical hernias.

Most small hernias of this type cure themselves before the baby is 3 years old. As the child grows, the defect becomes relatively smaller and unimportant. If this does not happen, a simple operation may be required later in childhood or adolescence. Larger umbilical hernias may require an earlier operation, if only for cosmetic reasons.

Note. Operations are not normally performed on young children unless absolutely necessary as the experience for a young child is a traumatic one. They should therefore always be delayed if at all possible until the child has reached the age of full understanding.

Exomphalos

In this more serious, but much rarer, type of umbilical hernia and in a variation of it called **gastroschisis**, most of the bowel is in a hernial sac outside the abdominal muscle wall. An urgent operation is necessary to correct the defect in the abdominal wall as soon as the baby is born. Exomphalos is often associated with other severe fetal abnormalities and is now normally detected during ante-natal screening. The severity of the accompanying abnormalities usually leads to the baby being aborted before it reaches full term.

Para-umbilical hernias

These are an *acquired* form of umbilical hernia which can occur in adults, i.e they are not present from birth. The hernia protrudes through a weakness in the abdominal muscle wall above or below the navel.

This type of hernia is quite common, particularly in women who are overweight and have given birth to several children. Para-umbilical hernias in this group always have a tight neck, and therefore there is a risk of strangulation of the bowel within them.

Incisional hernias

These occur following surgery to the abdomen in which an incision has been made. The skin of the incision heals, but the scar in the muscle layers becomes a weak point through which a hernia may eventually protrude. Sometimes incisional hernias occur when the stitches in the abdominal muscle layers give way. The skin which has healed over the wound remains intact.

Another major cause of incisional hernias is infection of the wound following an operation. It is also possible that post-operative bleeding in the wound increases the risk of this type of hernia developing.

> Catgut was once commonly used to sew incisions following operations in the abdomen, but it is now known that this material can cause a wound reaction, is rapidly absorbed, and can lead to the development of an incisional hernia. Except for the sewing of muscle-splitting incisions such as those involved in appendicectomy, catgut has now been replaced with synthetic, usually non-absorbable material such as Nylon to close the muscle layers.

Incisional hernias may become very large and painful, and can contain a large proportion of the gut. Small incisional hernias have a small neck, and therefore a high risk of strangulation of the bowel.

Obese people and the elderly seem to be more at risk of developing this type of hernia. In older, unfit people, a corset may help to control it, but this is never a very satisfactory solution.

Epigastric hernias

These are usually protrusions of fat which lie between the peritoneum and abdominal muscles. The hernia bulges through a weak spot in the midline between the navel and the breastbone. Occasionally epigastric hernias are large enough to contain a true hernial sac and abdominal contents. They are rare hernias – about 2% of all types – and are more common in men than in women.

Inguinal hernias

These are the most common of all, making up about 90% of the hernias which occur in the groin. They appear in the region of the inguinal canal as a swelling in the groin. They are more common in men, only about 10% occurring in women. Many young sports players develop inguinal hernias, which can be painful. However, the hernia may not be clinically apparent, and, rarely, may have to be demonstrated by **herniography**. (Herniography involves the injection of a dye into the abdominal cavity. If a hernial sac is present, it will fill with dye which can then be seen on X-ray.)

The testicles develop near the kidneys in a male fetus. They move down the inguinal canal as the fetus grows, passing through the abdominal cavity to the groin, and should enter the scrotum just before birth. In *indirect* inguinal hernias, a hernial sac containing part of the bowel bulges through the lower abdominal wall, following the track of the descent of the testicle. In young boys these hernias can be associated with an undescended testicle. They are therefore usually congenital, although the potential weakness may not become apparent until later in adult life.

Direct inguinal hernias protrude through the abdominal wall lining the groin, and are acquired. They are not related to the descent of a testicle, and are less likely to strangulate or obstruct.

Men may acquire an inguinal hernia as a result of hard physical work. Many report having felt a tearing sensation in their groin when lifting something heavy. Some people may have one on each side. Both types of inguinal hernia can also occur in women, but are much less common.

Femoral hernias

These also occur in the groin, but this time herniation is through the femoral canal, which runs alongside the main blood vessels in the leg.

Femoral hernias occur mostly in older women, approximately 1 woman in every 250 having one, or possibly two. They also develop in players of sports such as soccer, skiing, athletics, horse-riding and marathon running.

Femoral hernias can be very small, and are therefore sometimes overlooked. They usually have a tight neck and an associated high risk of strangulation of the bowel.

Other hernias

Diaphragmatic hernias are relatively rare and occur in the upper abdomen. The most common type is a hiatus hernia, which does not usually require surgery (see Chapter 11 for further details).

There are other rare hernias, such as *obturator* and *lumbar* hernias, which are beyond the scope of this book. They often become apparent as intestinal obstruction rather than as a lump in the abdominal wall, and are only discovered during an exploratory abdominal operation.

TREATMENT

> Note. A **reducible** hernia is one that can simply be pushed back through the hole in the muscle wall by gently exerting pressure with the hand. An **irreducible** hernia cannot be replaced in this way.

Although specific treatment depends on the type and site of the hernia, as well as on the age, sex and general health of the patient, some general principles do apply.

Not all hernias need treatment. Many can be left for years without anything having to be done, especially those occurring in the old and frail, and in young children for whom surgery would be a frightening experience. However, this is only true if the risk of strangulation or obstruction is very small.

For those who are fit for surgery, and whose hernias are likely to cause problems in the future, an operation is the treatment of choice. For people who are not suitable for an anaesthetic, such as those with a chest or heart complaint, non-surgical treatment may relieve the symptoms (see below). In some cases, the disadvantages of an operation may outweigh its possible advantages, and many people prefer to put up with the minor discomfort caused by some types of hernia rather than have an operation.

Symptom relief without surgery

Some simple hernias can be controlled by wearing a truss, although this is rarely recommended. In most cases trusses are inefficient and may even be harmful if worn on top of a hernia. A truss is a strap-like device worn around the waist and groin which applies a pad to the site of the hernia to prevent it protruding. Strapping may keep an umbilical hernia reduced in a baby but is usually used more for the parents' peace of mind than as an aid to the baby itself.

Surgical treatment

Of the approximately 95 000 hernia operations carried out in England in the year 1989–90, some 80% were for inguinal hernias.

Surgery is usually offered for reducible hernias before these can become irreducible or before further complications can arise. In time, the weak abdominal muscle wall may give way further and the hernia will become larger. Irreducible hernias are more serious, and should really always be treated surgically.

If your hernia changes from being a soft swelling which you can push back into place and becomes an irreducible, hard lump which sticks and cannot be pushed back, you must seek medical advice at once. Even if you are already on the waiting list for an operation, contact your doctor or consultant surgeon to describe the change in your hernia. Immediate surgery will probably be necessary.

Herniotomy

Surgical treatment involves reducing the hernia by pushing its contents back through the gap in the cavity wall. The hernial sac may then be opened to make sure that the contents have all been returned to their correct place in the abdomen, and then tied off and removed. This process is called **herniotomy**, and is all that is required for inguinal hernias in babies.

Herniorrhaphy

For other hernias, the edges of the gap in the abdominal muscle or connective tissue wall are then pulled and sewn together over the herniotomy. This repair technique is known as **herniorrhaphy** or **hernioplasty**. Sometimes, to avoid tight sutures completely, a piece of mesh can be sewn over the hernial defect to close the gap.

Laparoscopic hernia repair

Hernias are increasingly being repaired by laparoscopic techniques, also called minimally invasive or 'keyhole' surgery, which are much less invasive than conventional surgery. An instrument called a **laparoscope** allows the surgeon to see into the abdomen. It is introduced through a small hole which is made in the abdominal wall after the cavity has been inflated with a harmless gas, such as carbon dioxide. Other instruments are inserted through similar small holes made in the abdominal wall and through which the surgeon can operate. A patch of material is introduced to cover the hole in the muscle wall from the inside. (See Chapter 7 for a more detailed explanation.)

More detailed explanations of the operations to repair different hernias are given in Chapter 6.

WHICH HERNIAS REQUIRE SURGERY?

If the neck of a hernia is tight, it is possible that some part of the intestine, usually the bowel, can pass through it and become stuck. Obstruction or strangulation can then follow (see p.4). Most para-umbilical, femoral and indirect inguinal hernias have tight necks and are treated surgically for this reason.

Direct inguinal hernias normally have wide necks and therefore surgery may not be necessary as the risk of strangulation is low. However, an operation is usually advised. If not treated quickly, any small piece of bowel which becomes trapped and strangulated in a hernial sac may die and perforate, causing inflammation of the peritoneum – a serious condition called **peritonitis**.

If an incisional hernia protrudes through a wide defect and causes no serious discomfort, an operation will probably not be necessary as the layers of skin form a further boundary to keep it in place. A corset-like device may give some relief of discomfort. Closure of a defect of this sort may be difficult, and recurrence of the hernia is common. However, if the defect is small, strangulation of the hernia becomes more likely and an operation may be required.

Similarly, surgery for an epigastric hernia will probably only be carried out if there are complications or if the discomfort it causes becomes severe.

CHAPTER TWO

Deciding to operate

The decision about whether or not to operate is usually quite straightforward. If your hernia becomes strangulated or obstructed, you will need immediate surgery. If it is a relatively small swelling which causes you no real discomfort, an operation may be unnecessary, provided the neck is relatively wide and there is no risk of it becoming irreducible. Femoral, para-umbilical and indirect inguinal hernias are exceptions to this, as they protrude through a small gap and are thus likely to become irreducible, obstructed and strangulated. Although often symptomless, they are therefore usually treated surgically.

SYMPTOMS AND SIGNS

Symptoms are what the patient complains of, for example pain or vomiting. **Signs** are what the doctor looks for, such as a swelling.

The symptoms and signs associated with hernias depend on which part of the body is affected, but the main sign of a small, simple hernia is a swelling, which often only appears during coughing or when standing up. Normally a bulge will develop over a period of several weeks, but sometimes it can form suddenly – if you are lifting something heavy or straining, you may feel a sudden pain or tearing sensation. The area of the swelling may be tender and may ache.

Umbilical hernias

A small swelling, about the size of a grape, may be visible at the navel when the baby cries, but this type of hernia does not seem to cause any pain or discomfort. Umbilical hernias are quite common in newborn babies.

Para-umbilical hernias

These appear as a swelling to one side of, or above or below the navel, perhaps associated with abdominal pain. They can grow quite large, and are most common in overweight women who have had several children.

Inguinal hernias

The appearance of a bulge in the groin may be the only sign of an inguinal hernia. There may be an ache in the groin which increases as the day goes on. Discomfort may also be felt in the testis. Inguinal hernias are most common in men. They may become quite large and extend into the scrotum.

Femoral hernias

As already mentioned, these are often symptomless, although there may be a history of vomiting and pain. As femoral hernias are often small, they can be overlooked, particularly in obese people. They are more common in women than in men, especially in those who have borne children. They may appear as a small swelling in the groin on straining or coughing, but strangulation is often the first sign of their presence.

Incisional hernias

Incisional hernias usually show as a bulge along the line of, but underneath the skin of, an abdominal scar. They may cause abdominal pain, and occur most often in the elderly or overweight, in people who are not generally fit, and in those with diseases of the connective tissues. The most likely predisposing factor is a wound infection following abdominal surgery.

Epigastric hernias

These are not common, and are usually small, involving a tiny defect in the midline of the abdomen. They occasionally cause severe pain in the upper abdomen, and can occur at any age. Their symptoms may be confused with those of indigestion. Epigastric hernias are sometimes very difficult to diagnose.

On rare occasions, hernias can even reach the size of a rugby ball. A large hernia in the groin may rub against the thigh, causing inflammation of the skin. Large hernias may also make sitting down uncomfortable, and may make it difficult for you to wear your usual clothes.

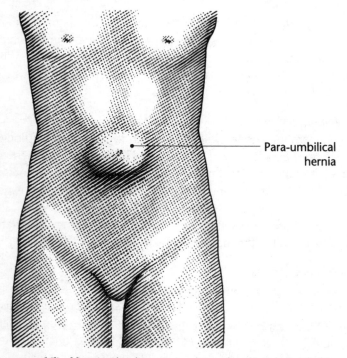

Para-umbilical hernia

A para-umbilical hernia. This diagram gives some idea of how large a hernia can become.

Young, and generally healthy, people are at little risk during an operation, and will probably be offered surgery, particularly if there is a chance that the hernia may become irreducible, with complications.

WHEN AN OPERATION IS INADVISABLE

Elderly people may not be considered fit for surgery unless it is absolutely necessary. Their weakened muscles may not heal well. People with chest or heart disease may also be unsuitable for surgery as they are at increased risk from the use of general anaesthetics. Local anaesthetics are used when an operation is essential for someone with these conditions.

WAITING FOR YOUR OPERATION

Once you have decided you want to have your hernia repaired, your GP will write to a surgeon at your local hospital asking for an out-patient appointment to be arranged for you. If the surgeon agrees that your symptoms are likely to be relieved by surgery, you may have to wait some time for your operation as simple, easily reducible hernias are not life threatening and the operation to repair them is not urgent. Chapter 3 gives details of some self-help measures which may be useful during this period.

If feasible, private medicine may be a useful option in this situation as it allows you to choose to have your operation at a time that is convenient to you (see Chapter 12). If you are being treated under the National Health System (NHS), you can ask for your operation to be arranged for a time that suits you, such as during the school holidays if you are a teacher. The hospital will try to fit you in as requested, although this is not always possible.

WHAT TO DO IF YOUR OPERATION IS DELAYED

If your operation is postponed more than once, or you feel that the length of time you have to wait is unreasonable, you can write, directly or through your GP, to the consultant whose waiting list you are on to ask whether your admission to hospital can be brought forward. However, the causes of delay and postponement of operations are usually outside the control of the consultant surgeon. If this proves to be the case, or you are not satisfied with the response to your letter, you can write to your local Community Health Council. Community Health Councils provide a link between NHS hospitals and the general public. They are there to protect your interests, and can contact the hospital on your behalf to try to find out the reasons for any delays. They may be able to reduce your waiting period. Your local hospital or Citizens Advice Bureau will be able to give you the address of your Community Health Council (see also p.136).

CHAPTER THREE

Self-help measures

The measures described in this chapter may help to reduce any discomfort caused by your hernia, although many hernias tend to enlarge over time, and surgical repair will probably be necessary sooner or later. (The self-help measures for hiatus hernia are different from those below, and are discussed on pp.91–2.)

1   *Try to control your weight*. Several types of abdominal hernia occur in people who are overweight. Weight reduction allows the weakened muscles to be strengthened by exercise and thus to provide better support for the abdominal organs.

2   *Try not to wear tight, uncomfortable clothing*. Braces may be a useful alternative to an uncomfortable belt.

3   *Try to avoid stooping or bending*. The intestines are squeezed as the body bends forwards, and thus the pressure inside the abdomen builds up. Part of the gut may then protrude through any available opening, such as a weakness in the floor of the abdomen or any defect in the diaphragm. **Try to keep your hernia reduced at all times.**

4   *Try lying flat*. Lying flat may allow a hernia to fall back through the gap in the muscle wall (thus reducing it), and can help to relieve its symptoms.

5   *Do not smoke*. Smoking causes coughing, which in turn increases the pressure within the abdomen and can lead to a hernia forming.

It is also important to try to give up smoking at least 2 or 3 months before (and after) your operation. Some surgeons will not carry out routine operations on people who have not been free from cigarette smoke for several months. Smoking also damages the lungs and arteries and puts a strain on the heart, increasing the risks of general anaesthesia.

6   *Try taking painkillers*. The ache or discomfort caused by a hernia may be eased by simple painkillers such as paracetamol; two tablets taken at night may be enough to provide a good night's sleep. If you are troubled by a constant, nagging pain throughout the day, you may have to take painkillers regularly during the day as well. If you are young and healthy and have never had any digestive problems such as a stomach or duodenal ulcer, you may get more relief from aspirin – a slightly stronger pain killer.

Painkillers containing codeine may also help, but these tend to cause constipation, which would further aggravate the problems of a hernia.

Whichever pain killers you take, do not exceed the dose stated on the container, and do not combine them with alcohol.

Be absolutely sure that any increase in pain, particularly if your hernia becomes stuck, is checked immediately by a doctor. Do not simply take more painkillers.

7   *Try to avoid lifting anything heavy*. Straining, such as when pushing a car to start it, or carrying heavy objects such as bags of cement or fertilizer, will tend to aggravate the symptoms of most hernias. If your job involves heavy lifting, do try to find ways around it. If you do have to lift anything heavy, use the technique described on pp.77–8.

8   Try to avoid becoming constipated. If constipation causes
     troublesome straining, the hernia bulge may get worse. If
     constipation persists, your doctor or pharmacist will be able
     to suggest many remedies to help you.
        **Persistent or increasing constipation, particularly with
     bleeding, should be checked with your GP.**
        A good diet of fibre-containing foods may help reduce
     any constipation. These foods include breakfast cereals (not
     only the high-fibre ones but also those such as Cornflakes
     and Weetabix), wholemeal bread, brown rice, wholewheat
     pasta, and pulses such as beans, peas and lentils. (Recent
     evidence suggests that fruit and green vegetables do not
     contain much fibre, although they are, of course, essential
     foods for supplying vitamins and minerals.)

9   Wearing a truss. Your doctor may suggest you wear a truss,
     particularly if your hernia is reducible (see p.10).
        The idea of a truss is to help to support the abdominal
     muscle wall and to push the hernia back through the gap in
     it. However, many doctors and surgeons do not advocate
     the use of trusses as they are expensive and rarely effective,
     and can also be quite uncomfortable to wear. Most feel that
     if a hernia is symptomatic, it requires surgical repair.
        A similar method of supporting an umbilical hernia in a
     baby by strapping is sometimes used (see p.10).

   Although many hernias may eventually require surgical repair,
the self-help measures described above can go some way
towards relieving some of the symptoms. If you continue practising these measures after your operation, you may also reduce
your chances of developing another hernia.

CHAPTER FOUR

Going into hospital for an operation

You should get a letter from the hospital telling you the date of your operation and any other details you need to know. Many hospitals also send out leaflets explaining the admission procedures and advising you what to take in with you. You may have been put on a shortlist so that if an unexpected gap occurs in the operating schedule, you will be asked to come in at short notice – possibly within a day or two.

LENGTH OF STAY IN HOSPITAL

An increasing number of hernia operations are now treated as day cases (see below). However, if you have other medical problems, or are elderly, you may need to have a blood test or other assessment, and therefore may be asked to go to the hospital a day or two before your operation, and be expected to remain until at least the day after it. Some surgeons still prefer all their patients to stay for a night after their operations. Whatever the planned length of your stay, you will not be discharged until it is felt that you will be able to cope at home. Medical staff may also want to be sure that you are able to pass urine spontaneously before you leave hospital.

DAY-CASE SURGERY

If, apart from your hernia, you are otherwise fit and healthy, the consultant may have suggested at your out-patients appointment that you be treated as a day case. Guidelines produced by the Royal College of Surgeons of England in 1993 suggest that 30% or more of non-emergency hernia repairs should be carried out on a day-case basis. The figure is currently nearer 7% in Britain, compared with 80% in the USA, but is increasing.

At current prices, the average cost of an operation involving an overnight stay in hospital is approximately three to four times greater than the cost of the operation done as a day case. Now that hospital expenditure is a major consideration, day-case surgery is seen as a sensible way of cutting costs and reducing the length of waiting lists.

You will be admitted to hospital an hour or two before your operation and will leave again a few hours after you have recovered from the anaesthetic. Patients have to be screened very carefully by medical staff to make sure that only those whose general health is good are selected for day-case surgery. People over the age of 50 are usually considered to be unsuitable for this type of care as health problems are more common in this age group, and therefore pre-operative tests such as chest X-rays and electrocardiograms (ECGs) may be needed. These tests are often done once you have been admitted to hospital, on the day before your operation, but can sometimes be done by your GP a week or two before the operation so that your time in hospital is kept to a minimum. Alternatively, the tests may be carried out on an out-patient basis so that your medical history, examination and investigations can be collated by a hospital doctor. This is called the 'pre-clerking admissions procedure'.

What to take into hospital with you

As you are unlikely to be in hospital for longer than a day or two, there are very few things you will need. The following list may be helpful.

1   *Nightclothes*. Loose, comfortable nightclothes are best. For men, loose pyjamas will be more comfortable after the operation, particularly for those with a wound in their groin. You will be given a hospital shift to wear during the operation itself.

2   *Slippers*.

3   *Dressing gown*.

4   *Towel and washing things*.

5   *Money*. A small amount of money may be useful for newspapers and the telephone. Large sums of money, wallets and handbags should not be taken into hospital as these may have to be kept in an unlocked locker by your bed. If you do have to take any valuables or large sums of money into hospital, you should give these to the nurse in charge of your ward when you are admitted. You will be given a receipt listing each item which should be kept safe so that you can collect your possessions when you are discharged. However, hospital authorities strongly discourage people from bringing anything of great value with them unless absolutely necessary.

6   *Books, magazines*. There will inevitably be periods of waiting between visits from medical staff before your operation, and you may want something to occupy you during this time. Apart from reading, it may also be possible to write letters or do some types of business work if your stay in hospital is longer than overnight.

7   *Loose clothing and shoes*. If you have a post-operative wound in your groin, this may be uncomfortable and clothes such as tight jeans will make it more so. Tight underwear should also be avoided. Casual, comfortable clothes such as jogging trousers are ideal.

8   *Drugs you are already taking*. Once your admission has been arranged, your GP will have been asked to fill in a form stating all the drugs you are taking and their doses. You may also be asked to take your drugs with you when you go into hospital so that their dosages can be checked and so that you can continue to be given any which are necessary. All your drugs will be kept for you during your stay as you must only take those which are given to you by medical staff. If you are asked to take your own drugs into hospital, these should be returned to you before you leave.

9   *Admission letter*. An admission letter will have been sent to you from the hospital, and you should take this with you when you are admitted for your operation.

Jewellery

Whenever possible, all jewellery should be left at home. Although wedding rings may be worn during an operation, there is a risk that any jewellery you take off before surgery may be lost or stolen. If you have to take any jewellery into hospital, it should be given to the ward sister for safe keeping.

Bleeding during surgery is controlled by **electrocautery**. An electric current is used to heat the tip of an instrument which then shrivels and seals the little blood vessels and stops the bleeding. Therefore wedding rings, or any other rings which are very precious to you or which cannot be removed, will be covered with adhesive tape during surgery as metal can cause electrical burns or electric shocks during this process.

Hospital staff

The ward of a hospital is a busy place and can seem rather confusing and frightening. It may help to have an idea of the different medical staff you are likely to meet, and the jobs they do.

Nurses

The uniforms worn to distinguish nurses of different ranks will vary from hospital to hospital, but all nurses wear badges which state clearly their name and sometimes their grade. There are, of course, both male and female nurses, although women are still in the majority. The nursing grades are as follows.

1   The most senior nurse on the ward is the *ward sister* or *ward manager*. Each ward will have one ward sister who will be very experienced and able to answer any questions you may have. The ward sister has 24–hour a day responsibility for all the staff and patients on at least one ward, for the day-to-day running of the ward, standards of care etc., and is ultimately responsible for the ward even when not on duty. The ward sister will be a registered nurse (RN), who has usually been qualified for at least 5 years. Ward sisters may wear a uniform of a single colour, often dark blue.

  The male equivalent of the ward sister is a *charge nurse*, whose rank will be clearly displayed on his name badge. Charge nurses may wear a white tunic.

2   When the ward sister is not on duty, there may be a *senior staff nurse* in charge. The senior staff nurse is deputy to, and works closely with, the ward sister. Like the ward sister, this nurse will be very experienced.

3   Each ward may have several *staff nurses*. These are registered nurses who have completed their nursing training. They may

be newly qualified or may have several years' experience, and will take charge of the ward when both the ward sister and senior staff nurse are unavailable. There are different grades of staff nurse, each distinguished by a different coloured belt, hat or uniform.

The more junior staff nurses are very often in their first or second post since qualifying. They are less involved in ward management, and are therefore able to work closely with the patients. Most of the staff nurses on a ward will be junior staff nurses.

4   *Enrolled nurses* are gradually being replaced. They have undergone 2 years of training and, like the junior staff nurses, are mainly involved in patient care rather than ward management.

5   As student nurses now spend more time in college and less on the wards of hospitals, *health care assistants* (HCAs) have been brought in to take their place. These are unqualified nurses who have undergone 6 months' training on day release while working on a ward and who have then been assessed for a National Vocational Qualification by senior nurses. Health care assistants are able to carry out all basic nursing duties except for the dispensing of drugs. They are supervised at all times by a qualified nurse.

6   The ward may also have several *nursing auxiliaries*. Nursing auxiliaries are not trained nurses, but are present on the ward to deal with any non-medical jobs and to help with the basic care of patients. Their duties include making beds, handing out tea, and putting away linen etc.

7   Student nurses – *diploma nursing students* or *Project 2000 students* – are unpaid, and allocated to the wards at various stages during their college-based training. They are mainly involved in observing, and carrying out limited clinical

tasks. In their last term before they qualify, they will be rostered on to nursing shifts and be part of a ward team.

The colours of the nurses' uniforms vary from hospital to hospital.

Doctors

Each consultant surgeon in a hospital heads a team of doctors of different ranks, sometimes known as a 'firm'. You may meet some or all of them. These doctors can, of course, be men or women.

1   The *consultant surgeon* holds the ultimate responsibility for all the patients on the operating list, and for the work of all the staff in the 'firm'. Consultants have at least 10 to 15 years' experience as surgeons. You may never actually see the consultant surgeon who is responsible for your care, but you will probably be visited on the ward before your operation by whichever surgeon is to perform it.

2   The *senior registrar* is a very experienced surgeon who has completed several years of training and is waiting for a post as a consultant. If your operation is to be carried out by a senior registrar, you may receive a visit from this surgeon on the ward beforehand.

3   Your operation may be performed by a *registrar* rather than by a consultant surgeon or senior registrar. Registrars have trained as surgeons for at least 2 or 3 years and are able to carry out some surgery alone, assisting the consultant, or being assisted by the consultant, on more difficult operations.

4   Some hospitals employ *clinical assistants* as surgeons. These are often very experienced surgeons who, for personal or family reasons, are not able to work full time. You may not meet this surgeon before your operation.

5   Before your operation you may be examined on the ward by a *senior house officer* (SHO), or, more probably, by a house surgeon (see below). Senior house officers have been qualified doctors for between 1 and 5 years, and are gaining further experience in hospital before becoming surgeons or specialising in another branch of medicine.

6   A *house surgeon* (or *house officer*) is likely to be directly concerned with your care both before and after your operation, taking notes of your medical history and arranging for any necessary pre-operative investigations to be done, such as a blood count, chest X-ray or electrocardiogram. House officers are qualified doctors who have completed at least 5 years of undergraduate training and are working for a further year in hospital before becoming fully registered doctors. Although house officers do not perform surgery on their own, they may assist the surgeon in the operating theatre.

Anaesthetists are highly trained doctors who specialise in giving anaesthetics and in pain relief. An anaesthetist will also visit you before your operation to discuss any relevant details, such as any anaesthetics you have had in the past and any drugs you may be taking (see Chapter 5).

Medical social workers

If any problems arise at home during your stay in hospital, or if you are concerned about being able to manage on your own once you return home, you can ask to talk to a medical social worker. Medical social workers work in close partnership with other medical staff in the hospital and will be able to give you advice and practical support.

For a short hospital stay such as is likely for a hernia operation, there is unlikely to be sufficient time for arrangements to be made for you to talk to a medical social worker while you are on the ward. If this is the case, and should you require immediate assistance on leaving hospital, such as 'meals on wheels' or a home help, the nursing staff can organise these for you, and can arrange for a social worker to visit you subsequently at home.

Procedures before the operation

Admission to the ward

When you arrive at the hospital, you should report to the main reception desk with your admissions letter. The staff there will check your details and tell you which ward to go to. Once on the ward, the ward clerk will deal with the clerical side of your admission, filling in the necessary forms with you. You will then be allocated a bed and introduced to your 'named nurse'.

The 'Named Nurse Initiative' was introduced into NHS hospitals under the government's Patients' Charter. A particular nurse is now responsible for planning each patient's nursing care throughout their stay in hospital. (The ward sister will, of course, still be informed of all aspects of your care, and will be able to discuss it with you or your relatives.)

Your 'named nurse' will admit you to the ward, look after you during your stay, and co-ordinate your discharge when the time comes. You will be allocated another nurse for other working shifts. The idea is for people to be identified as individuals who are known to at least one nurse on each shift and who are involved in their own care. To this end, you will be asked to help your nurse draw up a care plan when you are admitted to the ward. You should tell the nurse of any preferences or dislikes you have, for example if you prefer to sleep with several pillows, if there are certain foods you do not want, or if you have any ailments other than that for which you are having surgery, such as arthritis.

Your nurse's name may be displayed above your bed or on your bedside locker so that your relatives and other nursing and medical staff know who to talk to about your care. Your care plan may be kept at the bottom of your bed, but wherever it is, it is available for you to read. Nursing staff will tick off a checklist as they carry out the various procedures and will update the care plan with you as the need arises. For a straightforward operation such as hernia repair, the basic care plan will often be standardised, with room for adjustment to your individual needs.

Do tell the nurse if you have any problems or if you are anxious about *any* aspect of your hospital stay.

As you are admitted to the ward, the nurse will take notes of your personal details and explain the ward procedures to you. Your discharge will also be planned at this time. The nursing staff will need to be sure that someone will be able to collect you and take you home when the time comes. If this is not possible, hospital transport can be arranged for you. If you are due to go home the day after your operation, the nurses will have to be sure you can manage. The effects of anaesthetic gases, and other agents used by the anaesthetist, can stay in your body for several days, and although you may feel you are fully recovered, your reaction times will be slow and you may continue to feel sick and light-headed for at least the next couple of days. Elderly people particularly should have someone to help them for a day or two after their operation. All this will be taken into account as you and the nurse plan your discharge.

The nurse will measure your blood pressure, temperature and pulse. A sample of your urine may be taken for analysis to make sure you do not have diabetes or any disorder of the kidneys that would make the operation inadvisable. You will also be weighed as the anaesthetist may need to know your weight in order to be able to calculate the dose of anaesthetic you require.

You will be shown to your bed on the ward and told of any ward details, such as meal times, and where to find the toilets and day room etc.

Anti-embolism stockings

Once you are settled on the ward, the nurse will probably measure your legs for the stockings you will be given to wear during your operation. These **T**hrombo-**E**mbolic **D**eterrent **S**tockings (TEDS) used to be worn only by patients having major operations to help prevent blood clots forming in the veins deep within the legs as they lay motionless on the operating table, sometimes for several hours. However, they are now used routinely as a precaution in almost all operations, even those, like hernia repair, that last less than an hour. Although they may feel uncomfortable, there is no doubt as to their value.

The normal activity of the muscles in the legs helps to keep the blood moving through them. During long periods of bed rest or anaesthesia, these muscles are inactive and the circulation of blood in the legs slows down. A blood clot is thus more likely to form which can block the passage of blood through the vein. This is known as *thrombosis*. If pieces of this clot break off, they form *emboli*. Even one embolus may have serious consequences if it travels through the circulation and lodges in a vital organ such as the lung. Anti-embolism stockings improve the return of venous blood to the heart and thus help to prevent blood clots forming.

The nurse will measure your calf and thigh and the length of your leg, and will give you a pair of stockings of the correct size. Although you will probably be given these stockings on admission to the ward, you will not need to put them on until you are preparing to go to the operating theatre. You will be told to keep them on until you are up and about again after your operation – later the same day or the following one.

High-risk patients, such as those with a previous history of deep vein thrombosis, may be given subcutaneous injections of a low dose of heparin during their hospital stay. Heparin is an anticoagulant, found naturally within the body, which helps to prevent blood clots forming.

Visit by the house surgeon or senior house officer

As has already been mentioned, a house surgeon or senior house officer will visit you on the ward before your operation to take details of your medical history, including any allergies you may have and any drugs you are taking, and to examine you. Your GP may have already filled in a form giving the names and dosages of any drugs you have been taking, and you should have been told what to do about these. Do not forget to tell the hospital doctor of any other drugs you have been taking which your GP may not be aware of, such as vitamin supplements, cough medicines, aspirins etc., which are available from the chemist without the need for prescription.

If you normally take a contraceptive pill or hormone replacement tablets, you may have been told to stop these for a time before your operation. If you are still taking them when you enter hospital, for example if you have been called for your operation at short notice, you should tell the doctor. Contraceptive pills used to contain much larger amounts of hormones than do the more modern ones, and these high levels of hormones were sometimes associated with complications from blood clots. The newer pills are almost entirely free from these risks, but some surgeons still prefer their patients to stop taking them for at least a month before surgery. In some cases operations may have to be cancelled if this has been overlooked.

The medical examination is carried out by the house surgeon to identify any illness or infection you may have which could complicate the use of a general anaesthetic. If you are over 50 years of age or a heavy smoker, you will probably have to have a chest X-ray and an electrocardiogram so that any potential anaesthetic complications due to breathing or heart problems can be picked up.

The doctor will also mark the area of your hernia with an indelible felt-tip pen so that the appropriate site is identified for operation.

The house surgeon will probably also ask you to sign a consent form. Although it can be assumed that your consent to the operation is implied by the fact that you have entered hospital willingly, consent forms are widely used. By signing this form you are declaring that your operation has been explained to you and that you understand what it entails and have agreed to it taking place. You are also giving your permission for the doctors to take whatever action they feel to be appropriate should some emergency occur during your operation, and for any necessary anaesthetic to be given to you. Do read this form carefully, and ask the house surgeon to explain anything you do not understand.

Visit by the surgeon

The surgeon who is to perform your operation is also likely to visit you on the ward to check that all is well.

Visit by the anaesthetist

The anaesthetist will probably come to see you to ask you about anything that may be relevant to the choice of anaesthetic given to you.

Anaesthetics have improved considerably during the last few years, and a 'premed.' is now not always given routinely. If you or your anaesthetist do feel that you are very anxious and need something to relax you, you may be given some form of sedative, by mouth or injection, 2 or 3 hours before the operation. If you enter hospital the day before your operation and think that you will be too anxious to sleep that night, you can, of course, ask the house surgeon or senior house officer for something to help you.

False teeth

If you have any false teeth, crowns or dental bridges, you should tell the anaesthetist as these will have to be removed before you go into the operating theatre. A broken or loose tooth can be inhaled into the lungs during surgery.

'Nil by mouth'

This is a term which means that neither food nor drink must be swallowed. In order to prevent vomiting and the risk of choking on your vomit while you are anaesthetised, you will be told not to eat or drink anything for 4 to 6 hours before your operation, although you will be able to have a few sips of water with any tablets you need to take. If you are admitted the night before surgery, you will be able to have supper on the ward. If you enter hospital in the morning and your operation is to be that afternoon, you should not eat or drink for about 6 hours before-hand.

Smoking

If you are a heavy smoker and have not been able to cut down or stop altogether, you will be advised not to smoke in the hours before your operation. It is, of course, much better to stop smoking some months before surgery. The carbon monoxide contained in cigarette smoke poisons the blood by replacing some of the oxygen which is carried in it and which is vital to processes such as wound healing.

Obesity

Obesity also adds to the risk of anaesthesia, and for this reason people who are very overweight should try to lose weight before entering hospital. Indeed, some surgeons will refuse to carry out non-emergency operations on heavy smokers or obese patients as they consider the risks to be too great. However, starting a long, strict diet before your operation may also be inadvisable. The consultant will have assessed your weight when seeing you at your out-patients appointment, and will probably have given you some guidance at that time.

Shaving

Some surgeons prefer their patients to be shaved before a hernia operation so that they have a clear view of the area to be operated on. Shaving also makes the changing or removal of the adhesive wound covering after the operation a less traumatic experience.

If you have to shave, you will probably be given either a disposable razor or clippers. Although hair clippers are preferable, and prevent the skin being 'nicked' by leaving a layer of short hair on it, thus reducing the risk of post-operative infection, they are quite expensive. Disposable razors are therefore more commonly used. Occasionally, a hair-removing (depilatory) cream may be used.

If you are having surgery for an inguinal or femoral hernia, you may be asked to shave the groin area on the appropriate side. Men may also need to shave the top of their leg if there is a lot of hair there. For men who have a lot of body hair, and who are having an operation to repair an umbilical or epigastric hernia, the stomach region may also need to be shaved.

If you are anxious about doing the shaving yourself, do ask a nurse if someone can do it for you. Arthritis of the hands can make this a difficult task.

If your hernia is to be repaired by laparoscopy (see p.61), shaving will not usually be necessary.

WAITING

It may seem that you have been admitted to hospital unnecessarily early, and you may find you have to wait on the ward with little to do. Apart from having to be seen by all the medical staff mentioned above, who are responsible for many other patients as well, time will also have been allowed for the assessment of any medical problems you may have, and for the results of any blood tests to be received.

Sometimes operations are cancelled at the last moment. Although this is distressing, and can be very awkward for someone who has had to make special arrangements to come into hospital, it only occurs if an emergency has arisen. Other operations taking place on the same day as yours may be more urgent. If this does occur, you will probably be sent home and be called again as soon as possible.

You will probably be given only an approximate time for your operation, and be told if it is scheduled for the morning or afternoon. An operation being done before yours may take longer than expected if complications arise.

LEAVING THE WARD FOR YOUR OPERATION

Before being taken from the ward to the anaesthetic room or operating theatre, you will be given a hospital operating gown to wear and will be asked to put on your anti-embolism stockings. A plastic-covered bracelet bearing your name and an identifying hospital number will be attached to one or both of your wrists. You will then be taken from the ward on a hospital trolley.

CHAPTER FIVE

Anaesthesia

Y ou are unlikely to have talked to an anaesthetist at your out-patient visit, but you should be seen by this doctor on the ward before your operation.

An anaesthetist is a hospital doctor who has been trained in the special skills of giving drugs which cause loss of sensation or consciousness, or both (anaesthetics), and those which block feelings of pain (analgesics). Anaesthesia is a vital part of any operation, and a great deal of time and trouble will be taken to make sure that you receive the anaesthetic which best suits you.

THE PRE-ANAESTHETIC VISIT

The main reason for the anaesthetist's visit before your operation is to decide what type of anaesthesia would be safest for you. This visit also gives you the opportunity to discuss any problems or worries you may have concerning your anaesthesia.

The anaesthetist will ask you several questions about any anaesthetics you have had before, any drugs you are taking, and about your general health. It is important that you answer these questions as fully as possible. You should also mention to the anaesthetist if you have any false or crowned teeth, as these will have to be removed before your operation to avoid them being inhaled into your lungs while you are anaesthetised.

If you have had any problems in the past such as an allergy to a particular anaesthetic, it will be helpful if you know the name of the drug concerned or the hospital where the operation was carried out. The appropriate records can then be checked to make sure another type of anaesthetic is used for your hernia operation. You should also tell the anaesthetist if you know of any other member of your family who has reacted against a particular drug, as you may have the same problem.

The anaesthetist may also want to examine you and to look at the results of any tests you have had. There are different types of anaesthetic which can be used for hernia operations (see below), and some health problems will preclude the use of certain ones.

GENERAL ANAESTHETIC

This is the most common type of anaesthetic for a hernia operation. The drugs used will put you to sleep so that you have no feeling in any part of your body. General anaesthetics can be given in two different ways.

1   *Intravenous anaesthetic.* A general anaesthetic of this type can be injected into a vein via a plastic tube which is inserted into your hand or arm. It will put you to sleep within a few seconds.

2   *Inhalational anaesthetic.* This is a gas which you breathe in through a face mask. It acts within 1 to 2 minutes. As the use of a face mask can cause some people to panic, it is not normally applied until you are asleep.

During the operation, the anaesthetist will make sure you stay asleep by giving you more drugs as necessary.

Risks of general anaesthesia

People with certain medical conditions, such as heart or lung disease, may not be given general anaesthetics as they are potentially at greater risk.

Some people are afraid of being put to sleep by a general anaesthetic because they fear the possibility of never waking up or of suffering brain damage. Even today, with the tremendous advances that have been made in anaesthesia, this risk does exist. Although the risks of general anaesthesia are small, they do have to be borne in mind. If you are worried about this, you should discuss with your anaesthetist the possibility of having an alternative anaesthetic. (See pp.86–7 for further discussion.)

LOCAL ANAESTHETIC

A local anaesthetic is given by injection around the hernia. It blocks the feeling in that part of the body alone, by numbing the skin and tissues. Local anaesthesia may be combined with another type of anaesthesia (normally a general), and is given to relieve any pain that may be felt after the operation.

There are various nerves in the abdomen which supply the skin and subcutaneous tissues, and also the muscles of the abdominal wall and the peritoneum that surround the neck of a hernia. Local anaesthetic injected around these nerves will 'block' the feeling in the hernia and the groin for about 3 to 6 hours, thus relieving the worst pain in the few hours immediately after surgery.

Local anaesthesia can also be used instead of a general anaesthetic for people with other medical conditions such as chronic bronchitis, emphysema, or other lung or heart conditions.

Local anaesthetics on their own have also been used increasingly, and successfully, in recent years for the day-case repair of inguinal hernias. As they do not cause drowsiness after the operation, they are ideal for people staying only a short time in hospital.

There are very few side-effects associated with the use of local anaesthetics. Occasionally they do not block all the pain after the operation, and the anaesthetist will then inject some more anaesthetic or give you a painkiller, by mouth or injection.

Sometimes, the anaesthetist will inject the local anaesthetic while you are awake, and will then gently scratch the skin to make sure it has taken effect. Often the anaesthetic will not be injected until after you have been sedated, or it may be administered just before and during the operation to give the best control of pain. Whatever the method used, your groin will be numb for some hours after the operation.

Sites of injection

There are several sites for injecting the local anaesthetics used for pain relief. They may be injected a few inches away from the hernia itself. The nerves follow a predictable path through the body, and there are certain sites where it is convenient to block them. This type of block is called a **field block** because the injection is into several 'fields' of nerves around the hernia. Local anaesthetic may also be injected directly around the hernia to make sure that any nerves not caught in the field block are included.

SPINAL AND EPIDURAL ANAESTHETICS

These are types of local anaesthetic which can be injected between the vertebrae of the spine, into the space around the nerves in the back. They cause numbness or loss of sensation in the legs and groin which will last for 3 to 5 hours.

Spinal and epidural anaesthetics are similar, but a spinal anaesthetic will cause more, temporary, weakness in the legs and you will need less local anaesthetic. With anaesthetics of this type you can remain awake throughout the operation – although you will probably not be able to see what the surgeon is doing. If you are to have a spinal or epidural anaesthetic but do not wish to be awake, do tell your anaesthetist, who may be able to give you a sedative.

One advantage of anaesthesia of this type is that you will not feel any pain from your operation for a few hours afterwards, and are unlikely to need additional pain-relieving drugs during this period. However, its main advantage is for people with certain types of medical condition, such as lung or respiratory muscle disease or heart disease, for whom a general anaesthetic carries more risk.

OTHER MEDICATION

In some hospitals, a pre-medication drug ('pre-med.') is given routinely to patients to reduce their anxiety before an operation. A 'pre-med.' is given by mouth, as tablets or a syrup, or by injection several hours before the operation, and will probably make you feel sleepy.

You may be asked whether you would like to have a 'pre-med.', or you may have to ask for one yourself if you feel anxious and have not been offered one. You can, of course, also say that you do *not* want one if they are given routinely in your hospital. The anaesthetist will be able to discuss this with you.

If you normally take any other drugs, such as diuretics ('water tablets') or drugs to reduce high blood pressure, these may also be given to you before your operation if necessary. You must not, of course, take *any* drugs – including vitamin tablets etc. – that have not been given to you by medical staff, however innocuous you think they are. If you are concerned about having to do without a drug you normally take, do ask the anaesthetist about it

THE DAY OF THE OPERATION

You will be told not to have anything to eat or drink for at least 6 hours before your operation ('nil by mouth'). The reason for this is that any food or drink left in your stomach when you are anaesthetised could cause you to be sick and to choke on your vomit.

While you are still on the ward, you will be given your 'pre-med.', if you are to have one, and any medicines you normally take. You will then be taken to the operating theatre, probably on a hospital trolley. You may go first into the anaesthetic room or straight into the operating theatre to be given your anaesthetic.

The anaesthetist, or an assistant, will ask you several questions to confirm your identity and make sure that you are the right person in the right place. Your identity bands will also be checked. Many people have many types of operations each day in a hospital, and these checks, which may be repeated, are essential to make sure no mistakes are made.

The anaesthetist will then fit various monitoring devices to watch over you while you are asleep. A probe may be attached to your finger to measure the amount of oxygen in your blood; some sticky pads may be put on your chest so that your heart beat can be recorded on an electrocardiograph; and a cuff may be put around your arm to measure your blood pressure. All these monitoring devices enable the anaesthetist to make sure that the anaesthetic remains effective and that you remain well during surgery.

A plastic cannula will be put into a vein in the back of your hand, and any drugs will be introduced into your body through this.

Once the anaesthetist is happy with the readings from the monitors, your anaesthesia can start.

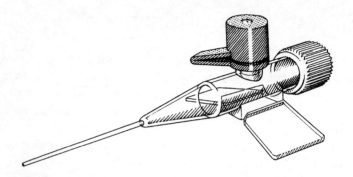

A butterfly cannula. This is an example of a cannula used to allow access into a vein, usually in the back of the hand. Drugs can be introduced into the body through this needle as required during an operation.

THE ANAESTHETIC

Whatever type of anaesthetic you have, the anaesthetist will remain with you throughout your operation, and may still be there when you wake up.

General anaesthesia

The anaesthetic will be injected into the tube in your hand or arm, and you will fall asleep within seconds. The drug which makes you go to sleep may sting a little as it enters the vein from the cannula, but this feeling does not last long. Several different types of drugs will be given to you to make sure you remain asleep. The following are used to anaesthetise you.

1   *Induction agents*: drugs which bring on sleep.

2   *Maintenance agents*: drugs which keep you asleep.

3   *Analgesics*: drugs which stop you feeling pain after the operation.

4   *Anti-emetics*: drugs which help to stop you feeling sick after the operation.

If local anaesthetic is injected into the wound during your operation to prevent you feeling pain when you wake up, your groin may be numb for a few hours afterwards.

Epidural and spinal anaesthetics

If you are having one of these anaesthetics, you will be asked to lie on your side so that it can be injected into your back. You will be told to keep very still while this is being done as the drug has to be injected accurately. The anaesthetic will take effect after 5 to 10 minutes; your legs and the lower part of your body will become numb and heavy.

You may be able to hear the doctors and nurses talking in the operating theatre, but the operation itself will be screened from your sight. Do tell the anaesthetist if you have any worries.

ANAESTHETIC FOR LAPAROSCOPIC HERNIA REPAIR

The surgeon may have decided to repair your hernia using laparoscopy (see p.61). Although the anaesthetic used for this type of surgery is similar to that for normal hernia repair, there are some important differences.

During laparoscopic surgery a harmless gas such as carbon dioxide is blown into the abdomen to allow the surgeon to see the hernia. As this is an uncomfortable procedure, a local anaesthetic would not be enough, and muscle relaxation is needed. Although spinal or epidural anaesthetics are feasible, the only option is normally a general if you are in good health. Your anaesthetist will discuss this with you.

One of the few disadvantages of laparoscopic hernia repair is that you may feel sick afterwards. This is because some of the gas used to blow up the abdomen remains within it for several hours, and it may also make you feel bloated and uncomfortable. The anaesthetist will use special drugs to prevent this sickness and discomfort until the gas has been fully absorbed by the body.

The incision that is made in the abdomen to allow the laparoscope to be inserted is small. Simple painkillers such as aspirin or paracetamol, and an injection of local anaesthetic at the end of the operation, will control any pain this causes.

AFTER YOUR OPERATION

When your operation is over, the anaesthetist will stop giving you the drugs that were keeping you asleep, and you will probably be taken to a recovery room or step-down ward.

The recovery room

The nurses in the recovery room are specially trained to care for patients coming round from anaesthetics after an operation. You will stay in this room, still watched over by monitoring equipment, until you are fully awake and ready to be returned to your own ward.

If you are in pain when you wake up, tell a nurse in the recovery room as you can be given an injection or tablets to relieve this.

The step-down ward

If you are going home on the same day as your operation, you may be taken to a step-down ward. The nurses on this ward will make sure that you are fit to go home and that your journey will be safe and pain free. They will also want to be sure that you have a responsible adult to care for you once you are at home, and should give you advice about how to manage your recovery over the next few days.

Back on the ward

If you are not going home the same day, you will be taken back to your own ward, where the anaesthetist will visit you before you leave. This visit is to ensure that you are having adequate pain relief and have no ill-effects from your operation. Do tell the anaesthetist if you have any concerns or questions.

SIDE-EFFECTS OF THE ANAESTHETIC

There are side-effects which can occur after anaesthesia, but these do not normally last longer than a couple of days. A sore throat is quite common, and is caused by the dry gases breathed while you are asleep, or by the tube which may have been put down your throat to help you breathe during your operation. You may have backache if you have had a spinal or epidural anaesthetic. Both of these side-effects will disappear within a few days.

If you feel unwell, or have pain anywhere other than at the site of your wound, do tell the anaesthetist – or a nurse on your ward – so that the reasons for it can be discovered.

PAIN RELIEF

The house surgeon and nurses on your ward will be able to give you analgesics to control any pain. However, if these drugs are not enough, do tell the anaesthetist or ward staff, who may be able to give you something more effective.

The amount of pain suffered after a hernia operation varies from person to person. Some people have pain or slight discomfort for only 12 to 24 hours and will not need any pain-killing injections after this. Others may need injections for up to 3 days after their operation. In the majority of cases, almost all discomfort will have gone by 7 days.

CHAPTER SIX

The operation

If you have had pre-medication, you will probably already be sleepy when you arrive in the anaesthetic room. The anaesthetist will then put you to sleep or insert an anaesthetic field block (see p.41). If you are having a local anaesthetic alone, which is most likely if your operation is for an inguinal or femoral hernia, this may be adminstered in the theatre rather than in the anaesthetic room.

Whilst the anaesthetist is looking after you, the operating team will be scrubbing their hands, and putting on gowns and gloves. At a minimum, the operating team will consist of a surgeon and an assistant, a scrub nurse, and another nurse to act as a 'runner' to fetch extra materials and instruments as required. There will also be an operating department assistant who will be there to help the anaesthetist and perhaps also to help with lighting.

IN THE OPERATING THEATRE

Once you are in the operating theatre, you will be transferred from the trolley to a soft operating table. Your thrombo-embolic stockings will be checked to make sure that they are correctly in place, and a wedge will be put under your heels to raise your calves from the table. These precautions are necessary to avoid the risk of deep vein thrombosis (see p.32). Anaesthetic lines will be attached to you, such as an electrocardiogram to measure your heart rate, a pulse oximeter to measure the amount of oxygen in your blood, and a diathermy plate for cautery (see p.25).

The surgeon will then clean the area around where the incision is to be made with an antiseptic solution; the light will be adjusted; and sterile towels will be placed around the part of your body to be operated on. If you are having a local anaesthetic alone, this will then be administered. When the anaesthetist is happy that all is well, the surgeon will begin.

INGUINAL HERNIA

There are several operations for inguinal hernia. All of them involve a cut in the groin which is usually made in a skin crease to give a less obvious, cosmetic scar. All the operations for inguinal hernias involve emptying the hernial sac, but for direct inguinal hernias the sac itself is not usually removed. For inguinal hernias in children, all that is needed is for the contents of the sac to be returned to their proper place within the abdominal cavity and, if the hernia is indirect, for the hernial sac to be tied off and removed by the process known as **herniotomy**. Usually a very small incision is made directly over the site of the hernia.

Repair of inguinal hernias

In adults, some type of repair is required in addition to the removal of the sac for an inguinal hernia. The operation to repair a hernia is known as **herniorrhaphy**. For both direct and indirect inguinal hernias, the repair is usually made using a non-absorbable stitch which remains in the tissues for ever. This closes the defect in the abdominal wall through which the hernia was able to protrude.

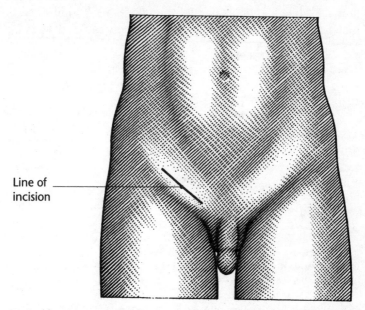

Inguinal hernia repair. This diagram shows the site for incision during the operation to repair a right inguinal hernia.

Line of incision

Once an incision has been made in the groin, the surgeon will open out the abdominal muscles to expose the inguinal canal which contains the spermatic cord and the hernia. The hernial sac will then be peeled off the spermatic cord within the inguinal canal. The spermatic cord contains blood vessels (including an artery and veins which carry blood to and from the testicle), and the vas deferens (which conveys sperms from the testis to the seminal vesicles). The surgeon will take great care to avoid any damage to these. As there is no spermatic cord in women, the hernial sac is easier to identify.

The deep inguinal ring and the neck of the hernial sac are then carefully exposed. If the sac of an indirect inguinal hernia contains parts of the bowel or fat, these are returned to the abdomen by twisting or opening the hernial sac. The sac is held in place while a stitch is passed through its neck. This stitch is then tied to prevent it slipping, and the empty sac is cut away.

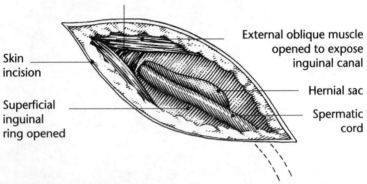

Deep inguinal ring where spermatic cord and hernia protrude from abdominal cavity

External oblique muscle opened to expose inguinal canal

Skin incision

Hernial sac

Superficial inguinal ring opened

Spermatic cord

Inguinal hernia repair. The inguinal canal has been opened to expose the hernial sac and the spermatic cord.

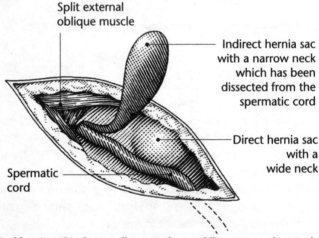

Split external oblique muscle

Indirect hernia sac with a narrow neck which has been dissected from the spermatic cord

Direct hernia sac with a wide neck

Spermatic cord

Inguinal hernias. This diagram illustrates the two different types of inguinal hernia which can occur – direct and indirect. The indirect hernial sac has been separated from the spermatic cord. The direct hernial sac can be seen in the background. These two types of hernia would not usually appear together like this, but can do so.

In direct hernias, the sac has a wide neck and the defect in the abdominal muscle wall can be repaired without the sac having to be opened or cut away.

There are many ways to repair the defect in the inguinal part of the abdominal muscle wall, the most successful being the **Shouldice repair**. This involves strengthening the connective tissue sheath which constitutes the posterior wall of the inguinal canal by overlapping it and rebuilding the deep inguinal ring. This repair is then reinforced by darning the muscles of the abdominal wall.

Another type of repair, called the **Bassini repair**, involves darning the muscles of the abdominal wall without first strengthening the sheath around the deep inguinal ring. The thread used in this case is a single strand (monofilament) of non-absorbable material, such as Nylon (much like fishing line), which is very strong and should last indefinitely.

The **Lichtenstein repair** involves sewing a plastic mesh over the weakness in the abdominal wall rather than stitching the edges of the muscle wall together. This operation seems to give good results, and has the advantage of being less painful as there is no pull on the tissues or stitches.

The external oblique muscle over the inguinal canal is then repaired using an absorbable type of thread. Sometimes an absorbable thread is also used to close the fatty layer under the skin before the skin itself is sewn just below its surface, with subcuticular stitches, to leave a cosmetic scar. The thread used to close the skin may be absorbable or non-absorbable; if the latter, it will need to be removed 7 to 8 days post-operatively. This method of wound closure gives good scars. The stitches are not visible on the surface of the skin, but the thread emerges at each end of the wound. Absorbable threads can be buried, but non- absorbable ones may be secured with beads on the skin to make their removal easier. Both types give good results, and the one chosen for you will depend on your surgeon's preference.

UMBILICAL AND PARA-UMBILICAL HERNIAS

Although umbilical hernias in babies do not normally require surgery, as they usually close themselves by the time the child is 3 years old, larger ones run the risk of strangulation if part of the gut becomes trapped within the hernial sac. (See p.4 for further details.) These, therefore, may need to be dealt with.

As para-umbilical hernias tend to have a narrow, tight neck, they often become irreducible, which may result in strangulation of the bowel. If this does occur, it can lead to significant complications. These hernias are therefore best treated surgically before they become an emergency.

Repair of para-umbilical hernias

An incision is made above or below the hernia. One above is 'frowning' in shape, and one below is 'smiling'. Once a cut has been made through the abdominal skin, the hernial sac and neck are carefully separated from the overlying skin before the hernia is opened. Any fat contained in the hernia may be removed. If there is any bowel within the sac, this is returned to the abdomen before the hernia is repaired. However, if the operation is being undertaken as an emergency, any dead bowel resulting from strangulation may first need to be removed. In this case, the hole in the muscle around the neck of the sac may have to be enlarged to allow the surgeon access to the abdomen. The sac, once emptied, can then also be removed.

The peritoneal layer on the inside of the abdominal wall is usually closed using an absorbable material. If the defect in the abdominal wall is small, the edges of the abdominal muscles can be brought together with a few large stitches. However, for larger defects, the abdominal muscle layer needs to be overlapped for greater strength, or reinforced with a non-absorbable mesh which is sewn across the gap. Both types of repair will be made with non-absorbable stitches.

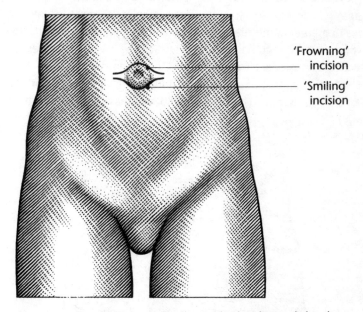

'Frowning' incision

'Smiling' incision

Umbilical hernia repair. Umbilical hernias can develop above or below the navel. A 'frowning' incision is made to repair a hernia above the navel; a 'smiling' incision is used for one below it.

The incision in the skin is then closed with subcuticular stitches, as for an inguinal hernia.

FEMORAL HERNIA

Femoral hernias invariably have tight necks, and strangulation of the bowel is therefore a risk.

Repair of femoral hernias

There are several approaches to a femoral hernia, the most common being from below. This operation can be done with local anaesthetic but the low approach is usually only suitable for non-emergency hernia repairs. A middle approach, similar to that used for inguinal hernias, can also be used for non-emergency operations. However, a third, high approach is used when the hernia is irreducible and strangulation is a risk, and particularly when there is a fear that dead bowel may need resection.

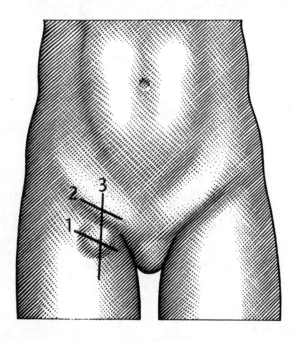

Incisions for femoral hernia repair. Incision 1 (the most commonly used, low approach) or 2 (the middle approach) can be used for a non-emergency operation to repair a femoral hernia. Incision 3 (the high approach) is necessary for an emergency operation when strangulated bowel may need to be removed.

The high approach involves making a long vertical incision rather than the normal small transverse one. This incision can then be extended into the abdominal cavity if part of the bowel has to be removed because of strangulation.

Once the skin has been cut, the hernial sac can be isolated, emptied and removed, and the peritoneum repaired. Two or three non-absorbable stitches are used to repair the defect, bringing together the lower edge of the muscle of the abdominal wall – the inguinal ligament – and a ligament on the pelvic bones. Once the defect has been closed in this way, the hernia should not recur. The skin is closed in the usual way, using a subcuticular stitch.

EPIGASTRIC HERNIA

Epigastric hernias are relatively rare and usually occur through a tiny defect in the midline between the umbilicus and the lower end of the sternum, or breastbone.

Repair of epigastric hernias

Usually an incision is made just over the defect. The hernia normally consists of a protrusion of fat which has pushed its way between the long muscles of the abdomen. There is therefore no hernial sac. The fat is not from inside the abdominal cavity, but comes from underneath the muscle.

The fatty protrusion is simply cut away and the muscles pulled together and stitched. Two or three separate stitches, or one continuous one, are made with a non-absorbable material.

However, if the defect is larger and there is a hernial sac with a wide neck, this can be inverted, as for a direct inguinal or incisional hernia. The muscles and skin are then repaired over the top of it.

INCISIONAL HERNIA

Incisional hernias always have a high risk of recurrence, particularly when the abdominal muscles are weak, for example in elderly or unfit people. Large incisional hernias have to be reduced and their contents returned to the abdominal cavity. This increases the pressure within the abdomen, which makes recurrence more likely.

Repair of incisional hernias

As incisional hernias always develop after previous abdominal surgery, the first step in the operation to repair them involves the removal of the old scar and exposure of the muscle edges of the defect. Some of the excess skin which occurs over the larger hernias may be removed. The muscles of the abdominal wall are then simply reclosed, using stitches of a non-absorbable material. To avoid damaging any adherent bowel, the sac is not opened but is inverted under the muscle repair. However, if the edges of the muscle have retracted well away, and if the neck of the hernial sac and the defect are large, a non-absorbable mesh will have to be sewn in place to close the gap in the muscle.

Finally, the skin is closed as for an inguinal hernia, using sub-cuticular stitches.

OTHER HERNIAS

There are other, rare, hernias such as lumbar and obturator hernias which occur in the abdominal wall. Some rare congenital hernias can also occur between loops of bowel rather than through the abdominal wall. These are sometimes only recognised when an exploratory operation is undertaken for bowel obstruction or suspected strangulation. This exploratory operation is called a **laparotomy**.

Laparotomy

This operation involves making a long incision in the midline of the abdomen to explore the peritoneal cavity and reveal the hernia. The contents of the hernial sac are then returned to their correct position, the sac is removed, and the defect repaired as in other hernia operations. Where bowel strangulation has occurred, this will also have to be dealt with before the defect is closed.

Note. Laparotomy should not be confused with **laparoscopy** in which a *small* incision is made so that a laparoscope can be inserted into the abdominal cavity (see p.61 for a more detailed description).

CHAPTER SEVEN

Laparoscopic hernia repair

Recent developments in the design of instruments used in surgery have enabled surgeons to perform a greater range of operations through multiple small incisions. This approach is known as minimally invasive surgery, laparoscopic surgery or, more colloquially, as 'keyhole surgery'.

The technique is now used routinely for removing diseased gallbladders and in gynaecology. The main advantages of laparoscopic surgery are an early discharge from hospital and a more rapid return to normal activity compared with conventional surgery. There is a cosmetic advantage as well. The single long scar of conventional surgery is replaced by several less obvious scars, each up to 10 mm (0.5 inch) long at most. The smaller wounds are also less painful post-operatively. The impressive results of this technique in gallbladder surgery have prompted surgeons to use it for other operations, including inguinal and femoral hernia repair. As the incisions made in the conventional repair of other types of abdominal hernia are small, laparoscopic surgery has less of an advantage in these cases, and so it is not yet generally used for these operations.

THE LAPAROSCOPE

The essence of minimally invasive abdominal surgery is the laparoscope. This is a type of telescope with a video camera and a light source attached which enable the surgeon to see the contents of the abdomen displayed on a television screen in the operating theatre. The abdominal cavity is inflated with carbon dioxide gas to provide space in which to operate.

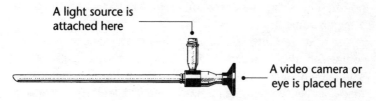

A light source is attached here

A video camera or eye is placed here

A laparoscope. This telescope-like instrument can be inserted through a small incision so that the contents of the abdominal cavity can be clearly seen on a television screen in the operating theatre.

An incision approximately 10 mm (0.5 inch) long is required to allow the laparoscope to enter the abdominal cavity. Specialised surgical instruments have been designed which can be used through small access ports (see below) and which are inserted, like the laparoscope, through separate small incisions in the abdominal wall.

General anaesthesia is needed for laparoscopic surgery, with the use of drugs which temporarily paralyse the muscles and allow the abdomen to be inflated. Other forms of anaesthesia are not suitable as breathing is made difficult by the inflated abdomen pushing up on the diaphragm and lungs.

THE OPERATION

Whereas conventional surgery for hernia repair involves opening the skin and muscle layers from the outside of the body, laparoscopic surgery is done internally, and the two techniques are therefore quite different.

The first step in the laparoscopic operation is to make sure that the patient's bladder is empty of urine. Usually a narrow, flexible tube called a catheter is passed through the urethra into the bladder to drain urine and to ensure that the bladder does not expand during the operation and get in the way of the operating instruments.

The next step involves inflating the abdominal cavity. A horizontal cut, about 10 mm (0.5 inch) long, is made through the skin immediately below the umbilicus, or navel. This incision is made deeper through the fat until the muscular layer is reached. A special hollow needle called a **Veress needle** is then carefully inserted into the abdominal cavity. When the surgeon is satisfied that the tip of the needle is correctly positioned, carbon dioxide gas is pumped gently into the cavity at low pressure. A special gas-delivery system is used to maintain the inflation of the abdomen at a controlled low pressure throughout the operation. Carbon dioxide is used because it does not support combustion and so will not allow electrical sparks from the cautery instruments (see p. 25) to ignite inside the abdomen. Carbon dioxide is not poisonous, and any gas remaining in the abdomen at the end of the operation is absorbed by the body and expired by the lungs.

After the abdomen has been sufficiently inflated, the special needle is replaced by a 10–mm tube called a **port**. The port incorporates valves to allow the continued delivery of the carbon dioxide and the insertion and removal of the laparoscope and surgical instruments without loss of the gas from the abdominal cavity. The surgeon will insert the laparoscope, with the camera and light source attached, into the port so that the abdominal organs and the internal opening of the hernia can be inspected.

Two or three other ports will be inserted through separate, usually smaller, incisions in the abdominal wall so that the surgical instruments can be introduced.

Repair of the hernia

Once the ports are in position, the hernia repair can begin. Various techniques have been developed for the repair of hernias, and the description which follows refers to the most commonly used.

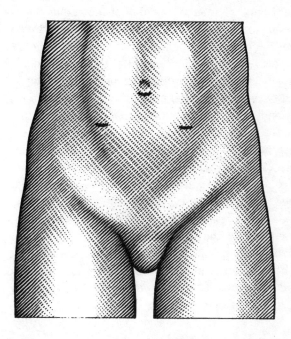

Laparoscopic hernia repair. Small incisions are made at various sites through which the laparoscope and other surgical instruments can be inserted into the abdominal cavity.

The hernial sac is emptied by restoring its contents to their normal place within the abdomen. The sac may then be removed by careful dissection, but not all surgeons agree that this step is necessary, and many leave the sac in position.

The peritoneum lining the abdomen is cut and peeled back from around the internal opening of the hernia. A woven sheet of special plastic mesh, which is strong and flexible, is used for the repair. The material is not absorbed by the body, and over time becomes incorporated in the fibrous scar tissue which forms around the hernia repair. The mesh is folded and passed through a port into the abdomen. It is then unfolded and positioned across the internal opening of the hernia. Special metal clips, similar to staples but which do not rust or corrode, or stitches are used to fix the mesh to the inside of the abdominal wall. This strong barrier prevents the abdominal contents bulging back into the hernia. The peritoneum that has been peeled back from the opening of the hernia is closed over the repair and prevents the abdominal organs becoming stuck to the mesh.

Mesh rather than stitches is used to close the defect in the muscle wall during laparoscopic surgery because of the difficulty of stitching from the *inside* of the abdominal cavity.

When the repair is complete, the carbon dioxide gas is released from the abdomen and the instruments and ports are removed. Finally, the small incisions are closed with stitches or adherent dressings known as Steristrips. Local anaesthetic may then be injected around the wounds to help to reduce post-operative discomfort. The catheter is removed from the bladder at the end of the operation.

AFTER THE OPERATION

During the operation, considerable swelling may develop in the groin and, in men, the scrotum may become very distended. This is caused by gas escaping from the abdominal cavity through the opened peritoneum and into the tissues around the hernia. The swelling has a peculiar 'crackling' feel, known as

crepitus, but is not painful or tender. The gas is rapidly absorbed and the swelling disappears within a few hours.

As has already been mentioned, the main advantage of minimally invasive surgery is the more rapid recovery after the operation. People having undergone this type of operation may be discharged from hospital on the same day, or on the following day, with almost no pain.

Full normal activity can be resumed as soon as comfort returns. There should be no restrictions on lifting or returning to manual work. Although individual variations are considerable, one or two weeks off work should be all that is necessary.

COMPLICATIONS OF LAPAROSCOPIC SURGERY

The laparoscope has been used by surgeons and gynaecologists for many years. Recent developments in video camera and instrument design have enabled its wider application.

Laparoscopy is a safe procedure, but there are complications which can occur, although these are rare. The main dangers involve the insertion of the special Veress needle to inflate the abdomen with carbon dioxide, although the surgeon's knowledge of the anatomy of the abdomen will ensure that the correct safe areas for this are selected. The Veress needle is designed so that a guard will spring forward to shield the sharp end as soon as it has entered the abdominal cavity.

However, despite care being taken, the Veress needle or port may occasionally puncture the bowel or a major blood vessel. The injury must be repaired immediately by opening the abdomen with a larger incision. It occurs in fewer than 1 in 500 operations.

Another possible complication during this type of surgery

involves the electrical cautery device used to stop bleeding from the little blood vessels. The heat generated by the cautery instrument can cause damage to other structures, including the wall of the bowel. However, this type of injury is rare.

LAPAROSCOPIC VERSUS CONVENTIONAL SURGERY

Minimally invasive hernia repair is a new operation and its technique is being modified as experience is gained. Although initial results appear favourable, no long-term results are yet available.

The recurrence rate of hernias repaired by laparoscopic surgery is not yet known, but evidence from the review of patients 1 year after their operations indicates that it compares favourably with the recurrence rate following conventional surgery. However, it will be several years before enough operations of this type have been performed to make a valid comparison.

Laparoscopic surgery has considerable advantages in terms of post-operative recovery and cosmetic appearance. For surgeons, who are familiar with conventional hernia repair procedures which have evolved over many years, laparoscopic surgery is a more demanding, time-consuming and technically difficult procedure. It will not be offered routinely to patients until surgeons are satisfied that it leads to a low hernia recurrence rate which is as good as or better than that for conventional surgery.

Authors' note

There is some controversy concerning the increasing use of laparoscopic surgery, mostly based on evidence from gallbladder operations.

Some evidence suggests that accidental damage caused during surgery with this technique may be twice as common as that associated with conventional surgery. A recent European study indicates that the figure may be even higher.

The benefits, both in terms of cost to the health service and less time off work for the patient, have led to a greatly increased use of laparoscopic techniques. The Scottish Office Health Minister has predicted that by the early part of the next century, laparoscopic surgery will account for up to 70% of operations.

The technique itself carries no more of a risk than conventional surgery; the problems lie in the training and experience of the surgeons who use it. Short courses of instruction in laparoscopic surgery are offered by trained surgeons in several centres around the UK. However, in America, studies show that the injuries caused to patients during laparoscopic surgery mostly occur before a surgeon has performed 50 operations using the technique. After this, the injury rate falls back to equal that of conventional surgery. Some patients therefore feel that they are being used as guinea-pigs on whom surgeons are practising and gaining experience.

There is no doubt that laparoscopic surgery performed by a surgeon experienced in its use is of great benefit. However, in the light of the recent evidence, you may wish to discuss the subject with your surgeon if there is the possibility that laparoscopy will be used for your hernia operation. Laparoscopic inguinal hernia repair does take longer than conventional operations, and may therefore be reserved only for bilateral or recurrent hernias.

CHAPTER EIGHT

After your operation: in hospital

Straightforward, non-emergency hernia operations usually last about 30 to 40 minutes, so you will probably be away from the ward for no more than a couple of hours. If you have had a general anaesthetic, you are likely to feel drowsy and slightly sick as its effects wear off. If your mouth is dry, you can take sips of water, but you should avoid drinking too much at this stage as it can make any nausea worse. You may be able to eat a light meal later in the day if you want to.

THE WOUND

Your wound will probably be covered by a clear dressing and can therefore be checked easily by medical staff. The wound is likely to have been stitched with a single continuous stitch under the surface of the skin which will leave a small cosmetic scar once it has healed. The stitch may be of an absorbable material that will dissolve of its own accord in time, and only its ends may be visible. Alternatively, it may be of a non-absorbable material with a small white bead attached at each end. Stitches of this type will have to be removed 5 to 7 days after your operation, and this can normally be done by the practice nurse at your GP's surgery or health clinic.

PAINKILLERS

A local anaesthetic may have been injected, as a nerve block or into the wound during your operation, to reduce the pain as you regain consciousness (see p. 40). Its effects should last for up to 6 hours. After this, and while you are still in hospital, you will be able to have pain-killing tablets or injections if necessary. Do ask for these injections if you need them, although regular oral analgesic tablets such as aspirin, paracetamol or Nurofen will probably be enough once any nausea has passed off, you are able to swallow, and your bowel is working normally. Make sure you have some of these tablets at home for the next few days. Pain killers should be taken regularly (every 4 to 6 hours, or as indicated on their container) so that their effect does not wear off before you take the next dose. A dose as you go to bed to sleep may be helpful.

GETTING OUT OF BED

Effective pain control enables you to get out of bed and to move around with ease soon after your operation. Movement and exercise are important at this time to avoid deep vein thrombosis and to keep your bladder and lungs working properly. You should be able to get up and walk about as soon as the anaesthetic effects wear off. You can then remove your anti-embolism stockings (see p.32).

Following an inguinal hernia repair, men may find it more comfortable to wear underpants which support the scrotum and prevent it pulling down on the wound, rather than loose boxer shorts or similar. These can also be worn under pyjamas. Men who have had a large inguinal hernia repaired may be given a scrotal support to wear before leaving hospital.

GOING HOME

Some time after your operation you will be visited on the ward by a hospital doctor to check that all is well.

Before you are discharged from hospital, the nursing staff will need to be sure that you will be able to manage at home. If you do not have help at home, and you are concerned about managing on your own, do tell one of the nurses *before* your operation so that some arrangement can be made for you. For some people, such as students who are returning alone to student accommodation, or elderly people who live on their own, a longer stay in hospital may be necessary until they are better able to cope.

You will not be discharged from hospital until your bladder is working properly again, any pain is under control, and you have no difficulties with coughing or getting about. Do tell nursing staff if you will have to cope with a lot of stairs or steps at home so that a physiotherapist can help you to practise with these before you leave the hospital.

Driving

You should not drive yourself home after your operation, and should probably avoid driving for at least 2 weeks. Your car insurance is likely to be invalid for at least 48 hours after a general anaesthetic: you may feel all right, but your reactions in an emergency would be slower than normal.

Even if you have not had a general anaesthetic, you should not drive until you are sure you can make an emergency stop without being hindered by pain from your wound, and are not a danger to yourself or to other road users. You can practise making an emergency stop in a stationary car but, if you are in any doubt, your GP will be able to advise you about this.

Discharge letter

Before you leave hospital you will be given a letter to take to your GP's surgery. This will contain a report of the operation and anything your GP may need to know about your treatment.

CHAPTER NINE

After your operation: at home

Once you leave hospital after your operation, you need to take a few sensible precautions. This chapter gives an idea of what to expect during your recovery. It also provides some tips on how to avoid putting strain on your wound as it heals, and how to cope with some of the everyday activities which may be awkward for the first few post-operative days.

THE LETTER FOR YOUR GP

The discharge letter which was given to you before you left hospital should be taken to your GP's surgery as soon as possible, preferably on your way home. Your doctor needs to know that you have left hospital, and to be able to make any necessary arrangements for your post-operative care.

The discharge letter will give your doctor the necessary details of your operation, and of anything else which may be relevant.

STITCHES

If your stitches are not dissolvable, you will have been asked to make an appointment with your GP or surgery nurse for these to be removed about 7 to 8 days after your operation. You should try to ring your doctor's surgery as soon as possible so that you can be sure of an appointment being available at the required time. The fact that your stitches will need to be removed will also have been mentioned in your discharge letter.

If you are elderly, or for some other reason would find a visit to the surgery difficult, ring your doctor and ask if a district nurse can come to your home to remove your stitches.

If your stitches are dissolvable, there will probably be no need for you to visit your GP at all, and you can remove the wound covering yourself after about 10 days.

Your wound should not be allowed to become soaked with water, and therefore you should avoid having a bath until it has healed and any non-absorbable stitches have been removed. However, showers are all right if your wound is covered by a waterproof dressing.

Some surgeons like to see their patients after the stitches have been removed. You will be told before you leave hospital if this is so in your case.

WHAT TO EXPECT

Pain

There is likely to be some pain or discomfort for a few days after your operation. Pain is the body's protective device to prevent you damaging yourself. You should therefore pay attention to it and rest when necessary. Painkillers will help to control any pain you may have, but do not let them mask this warning sign.

You may also have areas of numbness and tenderness, which can last for several weeks.

A few days after the operation, as the sewn muscle heals, you may be able to feel a ridge or bump under your wound, which is quite normal.

Bruising

Bruising often occurs following an operation and can be quite severe. It may not appear for a couple of days, and will probably last 10 days to 3 weeks. It is not normally a cause for concern, but if you are worried, do contact your doctor for advice or reassurance.

COMPLICATIONS

Complications can occur after a hernia operation and the main ones are described in Chapter 10. Knowing about these will help you to recognise when to seek medical attention. However, if in doubt, always contact your doctor for advice.

LIFTING AND STRAINING

You should avoid lifting heavy weights, including children, for about 6 weeks after your operation. Pushing or pulling, such as when vacuum cleaning, can also cause discomfort. If at all possible, you should try to get some help with these activities for at least a week or two.

A high-fibre diet is the best way to avoid constipation (see p.21) but, if this does not work, a mild laxative may be helpful to avoid straining. Your doctor will be able to advise you about this if you have any problems.

EXERCISE AND RESTING

Exercise is essential to avoid blood clots forming in the veins (see p.32). For the first couple of days after your operation, it will probably be enough to walk around your home from time to time, and to avoid sitting for long periods. After this, you should try to walk a little more each day, gradually increasing the distance over the next few weeks.

You may feel quite tired for a few days, and planning some quiet rest periods during the day will be helpful. Standing for long periods will also be tiring. If you cannot get help with jobs such as washing up or preparing meals, try to do these sitting down if at all possible. Bending and stretching to reach low cupboards and high shelves will also cause discomfort.

Getting up out of a low chair or sofa may be difficult for a few days, so try to sit in a high chair if possible.

DRIVING

You will probably be advised not to drive for at least a couple of weeks after your operation (see p.70). You should certainly wait until you would be able to brake hard in an emergency without causing pain in your wound, and can try this in a stationary car if in doubt.

RETURNING TO WORK

If you normally go out to work, your GP will give you a sick note to enable you to remain at home for 2 to 3 weeks. Some people feel able to return to office work before this time, although, if your job involves heavy manual labour, you will probably be advised not to return to it for at least 6 weeks. Contact your doctor when the time comes to ask for the necessary certificate to return to work.

How to reduce discomfort during normal activity

Simple, everyday activities may cause discomfort in your wound in the first couple of days after your operation. Anything which causes tension in the abdominal muscles can pull on the stitches, and, even if this is not painful, many people find it worrying as they are afraid they may re-open the wound. This is very unlikely, but the following suggestions may be helpful to avoid discomfort.

Getting out of bed

As you sit up in bed, the muscles in your stomach tighten and this may cause pain in your wound. You may find the following method of getting out of bed helpful.

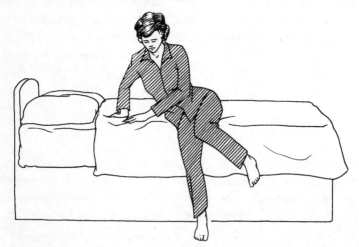

Getting out of bed. Once you have raised yourself from the bed, with your weight supported by your arms (as described in the text), you can gently lower your legs to the floor, one at a time.

1   Lying on your back, bend your knees up one at a time and put your feet flat on the bed.

2   Turn your head, and then your shoulders to the side so that you are facing the edge of the bed. Then, with your knees together, lower your bent legs to the side so that you roll your body over towards the edge of the bed.

3   Push yourself up into a sitting position, using your elbow and hand. As you do this, lower your feet to the floor, one at a time.

Coughing and sneezing

Coughing and sneezing can cause pain in your wound in the first few days after your operation as they involve tightening of the abdominal muscles. These actions will not damage your wound, but any discomfort that accompanies them may be reduced by supporting your wound with your hands as you cough or sneeze. Bending both your knees as you do this also helps to reduce the tension in the abdominal muscles.

Lifting

You should not do any *heavy* lifting for about 6 weeks after your operation. If you do have to lift anything, you should always make sure you use the proper lifting technique. This is important at all times, not just when you have had an operation.

1   Stand close to the object to be lifted, with your feet apart.

2   Do *not* bend your back, but lower your body towards the object by bending your knees.

3   Hold the object firmly and close to you.

4   Straighten your knees slowly and steadily.

5 Move your *feet* to turn your body once you are standing again. Do *not* twist the lower part of your back to turn.

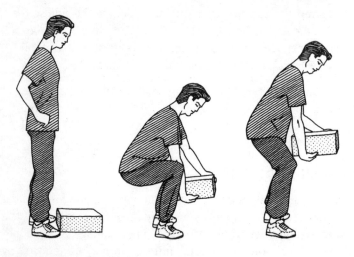

Lifting a heavy object. The correct lifting technique is important at all times. Having positioned yourself close to the object to be lifted, bend your knees rather than your back to reach it. Once you have grasped the object, straighten your knees slowly and steadily.

Posture

Any discomfort in your wound may cause you to slump forward or allow your back to sag, particularly when standing. This position will eventually lead to low back pain and should be avoided. Good posture will also improve the tone of your abdominal muscles as they help to control the position of the pelvis and therefore of the lower part of your spine.

When you first stand after your operation, take a few seconds gradually to ease yourself up straight. Always make an effort to sit and stand with your back straight, not slumped forward with your chin sticking out, and not arching backwards.

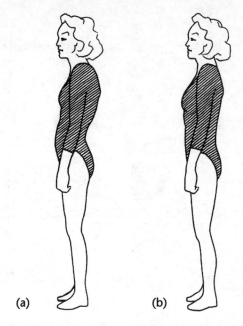

Posture. (a) Bad posture should be avoided, both when standing and sitting, as it will eventually lead to low back pain. (b) Good posture helps to improve the tone of your abdominal muscles.

Strengthening your abdominal muscles

About a week after your operation, you can start some gentle exercises to improve the strength of your abdominal muscles. But only do these if your wound is healing well and is fairly comfortable. The exercises described below can all be done on a bed.

EXERCISES

1   Lie on your back with one leg bent and one straight.
    Shorten the straight leg by drawing it up towards your hip.
    Repeat this 10 times with each leg.

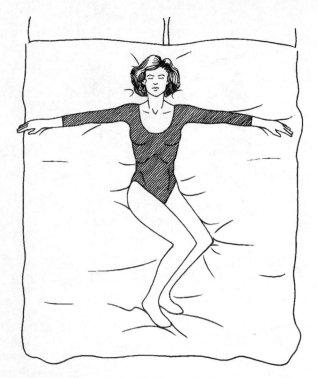

Exercise 2. When doing exercise 2, as described in the text, lower your knees towards the floor or bed as shown here.

2   Lie on your back with both knees bent and your feet flat on the bed or floor. Keep your knees together and, twisting from your waist, gently lower your knees towards the bed on one side and then the other. Repeat this 5 times. As this exercise becomes easier, gradually try to get your knees onto the bed.

3   Lie on your back with both knees bent and press the middle of your back down onto the bed. Hold it there for the count of 6, and then let go. Repeat 5 times.

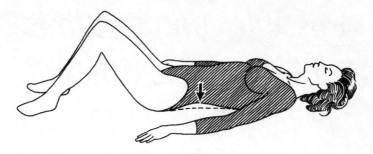

Exercise 3. Press the middle of your back down onto the floor or bed, as described in the text.

4   Lie with your knees bent and lift your head and shoulders off the bed, reaching your hands towards your knees. As this exercise becomes easier, reach towards your left knee with your right hand, and then towards your right knee with your left hand. Repeat 5 times.

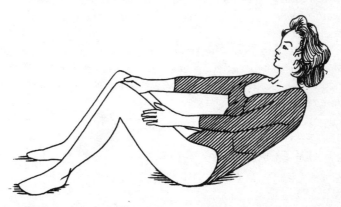

Exercise 4. For this exercise, lift your head and shoulders, and reach your hands towards your knees as shown.

If you follow the advice above, you should be able to do most of your normal activities without any undue discomfort.

81

CHAPTER TEN

Possible complications following treatment

All operations carry a small risk of complications such as deep vein thrombosis or a chest infection, and hernia repair is no exception. Precautions are, of course, taken to prevent complications such as these arising, for example by using thrombo-embolic stockings to avoid thrombosis (see p.32). There are also other possible complications which are peculiar to hernia repair operations. Although minor ones are fairly common, serious post-operative problems are rare. However, it is as well to be aware of what could go wrong so that you know when to seek medical advice.

The possible post-operative complications can be divided into those that occur soon after the operation and those that occur later, sometimes many years later. The early ones are more common.

EARLY COMPLICATIONS

Pain

Although it is normal to feel some discomfort in the wound after an operation, it is unusual to have severe pain. Post-operative discomfort can normally be controlled by simple painkillers, but pain after a few days may be a sign that an infection is developing, and if this occurs, you should seek medical attention.

Bleeding

There is often a certain amount of oozing of blood or fluid from the wound, but this is unlikely to be heavy. If oozing continues, and particularly if it leaks from your wound dressing and soils your clothes, medical advice should be sought.

Rarely, bleeding may continue and your wound may need to be explored at a second operation to tie off or cauterise a bleeding blood vessel which was overlooked during the operation or which has started to bleed again post-operatively.

Occasionally, bleeding which does not reveal itself through the edges of the wound may lead to severe bruising, which may extend down to the scrotum in men following repair of an inguinal hernia. Bruising may sometimes not appear until several days after the operation. Although distressing, this seldom requires treatment to release the blood which has accumulated under the skin.

Haematoma

In rare cases, a haematoma may develop. A haematoma is a swelling which is full of blood, and it is a complication which can occur after any operation, including hernia repair. The swelling is usually no larger than a grape, and is caused by a blood vessel continuing to bleed or re-opening after the operation.

A haematoma can sometimes be due to a disturbance of the normal blood-clotting mechanisms of the body. For example, drugs called anticoagulants are sometimes used to prevent blood clots forming in the deep veins, and people taking these drugs are more likely to bleed. There is a variety of inherited bleeding disorders, such as haemophilia, which cause a similar disturbance of the blood-clotting mechanism, but these conditions will be taken into account before any operation is considered.

Haematoma development is accompanied by pain, the formation of a hard swelling, and possibly a reddish purple discoloration in the skin. Bruising may appear around the wound or at some distance from it over the next few days. A raised temperature may develop if the wound becomes infected.

If you think a haematoma is forming or has formed once you have left hospital, you should contact your GP or consultant for advice. The haematoma is likely to be reabsorbed of its own accord within 3 or 4 weeks without the need for any treatment. If it continues to bleed heavily, with increased pain and swelling, you may need an operation to close off the bleeding vessel which is causing it. Your doctor may also wish to do specialised blood tests to check that your blood-clotting factors are normal.

However, you should bear in mind that some colour changes in the skin, due to bruising, are normal after most operations. These will disappear after a few days and are not a cause for concern, although their appearance can be quite alarming.

Wound infection

Infection can sometimes occur following hernia repair and is indicated by pain, swelling, heat and redness around the wound. As most modern wound dressings are transparent, it is now much easier to examine wounds for signs of infection.

Wound infection is slightly more common after surgery for recurrent hernias or after emergency surgery. When a hernia becomes strangulated and the blood supply to the gut within it is cut off, the wall of that part of the gut will die. As the gut wall is thin, its contents (which include bacteria) can break through and spill into the hernial sac and the open wound, causing a troublesome infection. Wound infection can also occur when foreign bodies such as suture material or mesh are left within the wound. Infections of this type are unusual, but may occur weeks or months after an operation.

An infected wound will become red, hot to touch, swollen and tender, and may be accompanied by a raised temperature. Pus or infected fluid may leak from it. Infection of this type may respond to simple cleansing of the wound, so you should seek medical attention if it occurs. Antibiotics given before or after the operation may prevent or treat such an infection.

In some cases, because the germs are likely to become concentrated around the stitches, some stitches may have to be removed to allow the infected discharge to escape through the wound.

Difficulty in passing urine

After an inguinal hernia repair, and very rarely following surgery for other types of hernia, passing urine may be difficult. Sometimes urinary retention is due to pain, but in older men it may be related to an enlarged prostate gland. If you are unable to pass urine spontaneously, a catheter may have to be inserted to empty your bladder for a day or two until the difficulty is resolved.

Constipation

This is not uncommon and should not be a cause for alarm. It may be due simply to the change of diet or reduced amount of fluid taken while you are in hospital, or to the relative inactivity caused by having to lie in bed. If you do suffer from constipation after your operation, it will almost certainly disappear once you resume your normal diet and activity at home. A high-fibre diet will be helpful (see p.21), but if constipation does persist, it may be with trying a laxative, a variety of which are available from any chemist shop. If in doubt, your doctor will be able to advise you.

LATE COMPLICATIONS

Recurrence

This occurs in about 1% to 10% of people following an operation to repair an inguinal or femoral hernia. The weakness of the muscle wall which allows a hernia to develop will remain after the operation, and therefore the original hernia, or a new one, may recur several years after surgical treatment.

The same predisposing factors which caused the first hernia to develop will also play their part in recurrence, for example smoking, coughing, heavy lifting, obesity and constipation.

Nerve damage

The nerves supplying the skin over the hernia are usually damaged as the skin is cut during an operation. These are normally only small nerves, damage to which will occasionally mean that a small area around the wound will be permanently numb. The area of numbness will decrease with time, but the sensation may never return completely.

Very rarely, small, painful and tender areas form in part of the scar, and this may be due to a swelling of the cut nerve ends known as a **neuroma**.

Nerve damage may lead to pain in the wound which will be relieved temporarily by the injection of local anaesthetic. Continued pain may respond to steroid injection. Only rarely is surgery needed to remove a painful nodule.

RISKS OF GENERAL ANAESTHESIA

The use of a general anaesthetic always involves a certain risk. Although the advances in anaesthesia over the past few years have been tremendous, complications still occur and, on very rare occasions, people do die during minor operations. Therefore, these small but real risks do need to be understood and considered.

If the supply of oxygen to the brain is interrupted during anaesthesia, there are two possible outcomes: death may occur without the patient ever waking up; or the patient may wake brain damaged and possibly paralysed. However, these risks are small: you are much more likely to be run over while crossing the road than to suffer any ill-effects from an anaesthetic.

Other possible complications are those associated with any operation and general anaesthetic. Immediate complications may include a sore throat resulting from the use of 'dry' anaesthetic gases or from a tube being put down your throat to help you breathe. A cough or chest infection may also develop. The muscle relaxants used during anaesthesia can sometimes cause muscle aches and pain, but these should pass off within 48 hours.

Careful consideration will have been given by the surgeon and the anaesthetist to your general state of health and all other relevant factors before deciding to go ahead with your operation and anaesthesia.

CHAPTER ELEVEN

Hiatus hernia

Hiatus hernias are diaphragmatic hernias, and present rather different problems from the abdominal wall hernias dealt with in this book. They are common, but rarely require surgery. When surgical treatment is necessary it is a more complex, major procedure than that for the abdominal hernias, and involves several days' stay in hospital. This chapter therefore gives only brief details of hiatus hernias and what you can do to help relieve the symptoms they cause.

WHAT IS A HIATUS HERNIA?

A **hiatus** is a gap or opening. The gullet passes through an opening in the **diaphragm** on its way down from the mouth, through the chest, to the stomach. The diaphragm is a thin, muscular sheet separating the digestive organs in the abdomen from the lungs and the heart in the chest. Immediately under the diaphragm, the gullet opens out into the stomach. The curvature of the dome-shaped diaphragm acts as a valve, allowing food to pass in one direction only – down into the stomach.

In people who are obese, or who have an inherited weakness of the diaphragm, the hole through which the gullet passes, which is normally about the size of a 50p piece, will gradually stretch and the valve will no longer work properly. Part of the stomach is then able to protrude through the hiatus in the diaphragm, and the acid which is present in the stomach and involved in the digestion of food can flow back into the gullet.

Unlike the stomach, the gullet is not acid proof, and the acid reflux into it causes inflammation and eventually scarring, as well as the chest pain known as **heartburn**.

Surgical repair for hiatus hernia becomes necessary when the reflux of stomach contents and digestive juices causes severe persistent symptoms despite medical treatment, regurgitation into the mouth, or inhalation into the lungs, sometimes leading to inflammation or even pneumonia.

Hiatus hernias can be acquired or congenital. **Acquired** hernias are **sliding** (90%), causing acid regurgitation and heartburn, or **rolling** (10%), causing discomfort and flatulence but without regurgitation of stomach contents as the 'valve' mechanism at

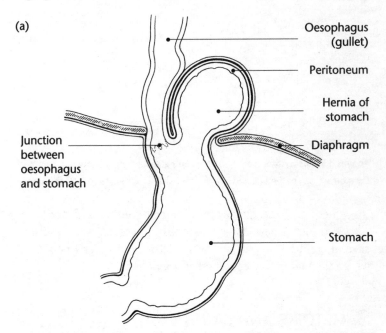

Acquired hiatus hernias. (a) In the less common, **rolling**, form of hiatus hernia the stomach protrudes through a hole in the diaphragm, causing discomfort and flatulence.

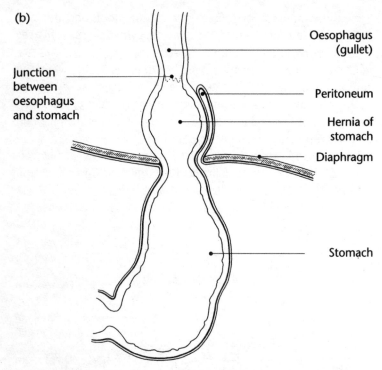

(b)

Oesophagus (gullet)

Junction between oesophagus and stomach

Peritoneum

Hernia of stomach

Diaphragm

Stomach

Acquired hiatus hernias (cont.). (b) In a **sliding** hiatus hernia, the acid contents of the stomach can be regurgitated into the oesophagus, causing severe heartburn.

the junction of the gullet and stomach continues to function. Acquired hiatus hernias usually occur in women who have had several children or who are overweight, or in elderly people in whom the hiatus has weakened and widened.

SYMPTOMS AND SIGNS

Hiatus hernias often cause only mild indigestion and are therefore ignored, only being revealed on X-rays for other conditions.

They are commonly associated with inflammation of the gullet or oesophagus, known as **reflux oesophagitis**. Oesophagitis is felt as the burning sensation of heartburn behind the breast-bone which can be confused with the pain of heart problems such as angina or even a heart attack.

The oesophagitis resulting from a hiatus hernia may also cause painful spasms of the oesophagus and difficulty in swallowing. Over many years, the acid burning the bottom of the gullet can cause scars to form. As these scars shrink, the gullet becomes narrower, causing a stricture which makes swallowing difficult and results in discomfort as food becomes stuck in the gullet above the opening to the stomach. When the condition is as severe as this, surgery is almost always necessary.

NON-OPERATIVE TREATMENT

Where symptoms do occur, they may be relieved in the following ways.

1   Simple measures such as *losing weight* may completely relieve the symptoms of belching, regurgitation and burning.

2   Some of the symptoms can be improved by trying to *avoid bending and stooping*, as these actions often cause the acid to pour from the stomach into the gullet.

3   Heartburn which wakes you while sleeping can be helped by *lying propped up* on several pillows. This is because lying flat allows the acid contents of the stomach to flow more easily into the gullet. Although in severe cases this symptom may be relieved by sleeping in an armchair, it is important that you do *not* do this if you are elderly or have heart disease as it can cause swelling of the legs as fluid, which can no longer drain away, accumulates in the ankles. This accumulation of fluid can aggravate heart failure in the elderly.

4   In recent years, many *drugs* have been developed which
     reduce or entirely stop the acid production from the
     stomach. Surprisingly, this does not appear to have any
     adverse effects on digestion. These drugs can bring
     immense relief to people troubled by the persistent pain of
     heartburn. However, less expensive, simple antacids may be
     equally effective.

     Other drugs are also available which improve the
     contractions of the gullet, help ease the painful spasms that
     can occur, or help to protect the gullet from acid reflux.

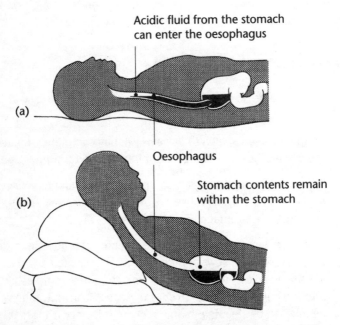

Acidic fluid from the stomach
can enter the oesophagus

(a)

Oesophagus

Stomach contents remain
within the stomach

(b)

Relieving the symptoms of heartburn caused by a hiatus hernia. (a) When
lying flat, acidic fluid from the stomach enters into the oesophagus as shown in
this diagram, causing irritation and inflammation. (b) With the head raised on
pillows, the fluid is more likely to remain in the stomach.

Your doctor will be able to advise you of the best way to deal with the symptoms of your hiatus hernia. If surgery does become necessary, you should ask for a full explanation of what this will involve.

CHAPTER TWELVE

Private care

There are various reasons why people choose to have their operations done privately. They may have private health insurance, or be covered by a private health scheme run by the company for which they work, or they may be able to pay for private care themselves. Whatever your situation, you will not find that the *standard* of medical care you receive in a private hospital is any different from that available on the National Health Service (NHS). However, you may prefer the privacy of a private hospital; or you may find the much-reduced waiting time to see a consultant, and to enter hospital for your operation, is more convenient for you.

The information given in other chapters in this book is equally relevant whichever system you choose. This chapter deals with those aspects of private health care which differ from those of the NHS.

PRIVATE HEALTH INSURANCE

If the company you work for has a private health insurance scheme, your Company Secretary will be able to give you details, and should be able to tell you if the company insurance covers you for an operation to repair a hernia.

If you have your own health insurance with one of the many insurance companies which deal with this, they will be able to let you know exactly what is covered by your particular policy, if this is not clear from the literature you already have.

There are different levels of health insurance, and you need to check your policy carefully to make sure you know what costs are covered. Most private hospitals have an administration officer who will check your policy for you if you are in any doubt. The staff at the hospital are likely to be very helpful and will try to sort out any problems and queries you have. But do read your policy carefully, and any information sent to you by the hospital, as unexpected charges, such as consultants' fees that you thought were covered by your insurance policy, could add up to quite a lot of money.

With some types of private health insurance, you will need to ask your GP to fill in a form stating that your operation is necessary and cannot be done in an NHS hospital within a certain time period due to long waiting lists. You will have to pay your GP for this service, which will cost a few pounds. This money is not redeemable from your insurers.

FIXED PRICE CARE

You may be in the position of being able to pay to have your operation done privately. The Bookings Manager at a private hospital will be able to give you an idea of the cost involved. Some private hospitals run a service known as Fixed Price Care: a price can be quoted to you before you enter hospital which covers the cost of your operation and a variety of other hospitalisation costs. You should always ask to have the quotation in writing *before* you enter hospital, with a written note of all the costs it covers. At some hospitals, the fixed price will include accommodation, nursing, meals, drugs, dressings, operating theatre fees, X-rays etc. At others only some of these costs are included. Once you have a quotation of this sort, you should not have to worry about any hidden costs that you had not accounted for. However, the price quoted to you by the hospital may not include the fees of the consultant surgeon or consultant anaesthetist, and you may have to ask your consultant for a note of these.

With Fixed Price Care, all the hospitalisation costs included by that particular hospital are covered should you need to stay longer than expected in hospital (usually up to a maximum of 28 days) as a direct result of complications arising from your original reason for admission – i.e. your hernia. In other words, if you develop some problem while in hospital that is unrelated to the hernia, the price you have been quoted will not cover treatment to deal with this. If, on the other hand, you should have heavy bleeding post-operatively, or some other complication which makes your consultant decide to keep you in hospital for longer than originally planned, all the costs that arise from your stay and are included in the hospital's fixed price (again, with the possible exception of consultants' fees) will be covered. At some hospitals, the quoted price will also cover your treatment should you have to be re-admitted due to a complication related to your original operation and arising within a limited period of time after your original discharge.

The only extra charges that you will have to pay to the hospital will probably include those for telephone calls, any alcohol if you have this with your meals, food provided for your visitors, personal laundry done by the hospital, hairdressing, and for any similar items such as you would have to pay for in a hotel. It is usually possible for a visitor to eat meals with you in your room, and for tea and snacks to be ordered for visitors during the day. (You will also have to pay these extra charges before you leave the hospital if you are being treated under private health insurance.) It is important therefore that you ask in advance for written confirmation of the price you will have to pay for your stay in hospital and what is included in the quotation. If the hospital does not have a Fixed Price Care or similar system in use, make sure that all possible costs are listed.

ARRANGING THE OPERATION

Although the medical treatment you receive in a private hospital will be similar to that available at any NHS hospital, there are some basic differences between the two systems.

As with the NHS, you will have to be referred to a consultant by your GP. Most GPs have contacts with particular consultants (and private hospitals) to whom they tend to refer patients. If there is a private hospital you particularly want to go to, or a consultant you have some reason to prefer, you can ask your GP to make an appointment for you.

After your visit to your GP, you are unlikely to have to wait longer than a week or two before you see the consultant at an out-patient appointment. Your appointment may be at the private hospital where your operation is to be carried out, at an NHS hospital which has private wards, or at the consultant's private consulting rooms. Once the consultant has agreed to operate, you will probably be able to enter hospital within another week. If there is some reason why you want your operation to be done even sooner than this, for example if you have to go abroad, this can usually be arranged.

If you do not have private health insurance and the hospital's fixed price scheme does not cover consultants' fees, you should ask your consultant exactly how much you will have to pay for his or her fees and for those of the anaesthetist. There are anaesthetists on most consultants' teams who carry out private operations with them.

Once your consultant has arranged with the hospital for your operation to take place, you will receive confirmation of this from the Bookings Manager of the hospital you are to attend. You will also probably be sent leaflets and any further relevant details of how to prepare for your entry to hospital. Do read these carefully, as knowing how your particular hospital organises things will help you to be prepared when you arrive for your operation. You will also be sent a **pre-admission form** to fill in and take with you when you go for your operation.

If your operation is being paid for by insurance, you will be asked to take a completed insurance form with you when you are admitted to hospital. You should have been given some of these forms when you first took out your policy, but your insurance company will be able to supply the correct form if you have any problems. If you are covered by company insurance, the form will probably be filled in and given to you by your Company Secretary.

ADMISSION TO HOSPITAL

When you arrive at the hospital, the receptionist will contact the admissions department, and a ward receptionist will come to collect you. If you are paying for your stay in hospital yourself, you will probably be asked to pay your bill in advance at this stage if you have not already done so. The ward receptionist will take you to your room – probably a single or double room – and show you the facilities available there. You may have a private bathroom, a television, and a telephone by your bed. The ward receptionist will explain hospital procedures to you, and will leave you to settle in. You will probably be asked for your completed insurance form, if relevant.

A member of the nursing staff will then come to make a note of your medical details, in much the same way as described in Chapter 4. The main difference you are likely to notice if you have been treated in an NHS hospital before, is that this time there is much less waiting for all the routine hospital procedures to be dealt with. The nurse to patient ratio is higher in private hospitals and so someone is usually available to deal with the pre-operative procedures quite quickly.

Although fully qualified doctors will always be available in the hospital, it will be your own consultant who deals with your medical care throughout your stay. Your consultant will visit you before the operation, will perform the operation (with the assistance of the anaesthetist and the operating staff), and will visit you again when you are back in your own room. Trainees - whether doctors or nurses – do not work in private hospitals. The consultants are responsible for their own patients and supervise their care themselves. Most private hospitals now have resident medical officers – fully qualified, registered doctors who are available 24 hours a day to deal with any emergencies which may arise.

PREPARING FOR YOUR OPERATION

When the time for your operation approaches, a porter and nurse will take you from your room to the anaesthetic room. In many private hospitals, you will not be moved from your bed onto a trolley until you have been anaesthetised; the bed itself will be wheeled from your room. Similarly, you will be transferred back from the trolley to your own bed in the recovery room while you are still asleep. You therefore go to sleep and wake up in your own hospital bed.

The operation will be carried out in the same way as described in Chapter 6. When you are fully awake, you will be taken back to your room to rest.

DISCHARGE FROM HOSPITAL

When you are ready to be discharged from hospital, the ward receptionist will ask you to pay any outstanding charges not covered by the hospitalisation charge. You will be given any medical items you may need from the hospital pharmacy.

DIFFERENCES AND SIMILARITIES

The main aim of the staff of any private hospital is the same as that in an NHS hospital – to make your stay as pleasant and as comfortable as possible. Because the staffing ratio is higher in private hospitals, more emphasis can be placed on privacy and comfort.

The consultant surgeons and anaesthetists who work in private hospitals almost always work in an NHS hospital as well, so you will receive the same expertise and skill under both systems. However, in an NHS hospital you may not actually be operated on by the consultant surgeon who heads the surgical team, and, indeed, you may not see the consultant at all during your hospital stay.

Private hospitals arrange their operating lists differently from NHS hospitals. The NHS hospitals have 'sessional bookings' for their operating theatres. This means a particular day is set aside at regular intervals for a specialist in one type of surgery to perform operations. In private hospitals, the consultants can book the use of an operating theatre (and the assistance of the staff who work in it) on any day, at any time that suits them and their patients. Therefore, your operation can take place privately with minimum delay, and at a time that is convenient to you and your consultant.

It is also possible, even if you are already on an NHS waiting list, to tell your GP or consultant at any time that you would like to change to private care. If the consultant you have already seen under the NHS does not have a private practice, you can ask your GP to put you in touch with a consultant who *can* see you privately. It is, however, advisable to find out how much private care is likely to cost before your name is taken off the NHS waiting list.

Summary

There are several reasons why, if they can, some people may choose to have their hernia repair operations done privately, either paid for by private health insurance or from their own pockets. Some people find it much more convenient to be able to have a say in when their operation is to take place. The NHS, under which the majority of people are treated, naturally has longer waiting lists. A routine operation to repair a hernia is not an emergency, and therefore you will not be placed at the top of the waiting list for your operation to be done on the NHS. If time is an important factor for you, you may be happy to pay to have your operation done at a time that you find convenient. Some people simply prefer the smaller, more intimate setting they are likely to find in a private hospital. Private hospitals rarely deal with accidents and emergency treatment; the operations carried out in them are normally planned, at least a day or two in advance. Therefore, they do not have the bustle of an NHS hospital which has to deal with emergency admissions as well as the routine admissions for non-emergency operations.

Questions and answers

The answers to most of the questions below can be found elsewhere in this book. However, you may find this section helpful in compiling your own list of questions to ask your GP or consultant. It is useful to write down questions as they occur to you, and to take your list with you to your doctor's appointment. Most people find it difficult to remember the things they want to ask when they are trying to take in the information being given to them by their doctor.

The answers given here are general, and your GP or surgeon may have slightly different information to give you, depending on what happens at your particular hospital. Do ask your GP, the hospital doctor who is in charge of your care, or a member of the nursing staff if there is anything you do not understand. No question is too trivial, particularly if it concerns something that is worrying you.

1. My GP is making an appointment for me to see a consultant at the hospital. How long will I have to wait?

This will depend partly on the severity of the symptoms caused by your hernia. If it is very painful and is making your life difficult, your GP will have mentioned this in the letter to the consultant. The consultant may be able to fit your appointment in at short notice – possibly within 2 or 3 weeks.

If your hernia does not require urgent treatment, you may have to wait several weeks before your out-patients appointment. Waiting lists vary between areas as well as between consultants.

If you are on a long waiting list and your pain is increasing, you can ask your GP to make an appointment with another consultant who may have a shorter list. Do not suffer in silence, and do not be afraid to 'pester' your doctor!

2.   The consultant surgeon has agreed to operate. How long will it be before I am admitted to hospital?

Again, you may have to wait anything from a couple of weeks to a year or more. You can ask to be put on a standby list, which means you may be called at short notice if a gap appears on the waiting list. You will then have to be prepared to enter hospital within a couple of days of being contacted.

The lengths of waiting lists for operations also vary from region to region. It may be worth asking if your GP knows how long patients tend to have to wait to see your particular consultant.

If your hernia worsens, do contact your GP again, and ask if another letter can be written to the consultant.

3.   I am on a waiting list, and have been told that my operation is likely to be within a couple of months. However, my hernia has become more painful recently, and it is now a hard lump which I can no longer push back. What should I do?

Contact your doctor immediately. Your hernia may have become strangulated and the gut trapped within it may die if it is not treated as a matter of urgency. Your doctor may arrange for you to be admitted to hospital as an emergency, and you may have an operation shortly afterwards.

4.   My GP recently diagnosed a para-umbilical hernia, and I am waiting to see a consultant. Over the last few days I have started to feel sick and generally unwell. My stomach has swollen and I get occasional painful griping pains. Should I just wait for my appointment to come through?

No. Your hernia may have become obstructed and, if so, food will eventually not be able to pass through your intestines. You should contact your doctor immediately as you will need urgent treatment if obstruction has occurred.

5.   I am 58 years old and have a small, irritating inguinal hernia. I am afraid that this will get worse over the next few years, and that eventually I will be too old for surgery to be a safe option. I would therefore like to have it treated now, but the consultant I have seen was reluctant to consider an operation. I am a heavy smoker, but rarely have any chest complaints. Might the surgeon change his mind and agree to surgery?

There are several factors which need careful consideration here, and your consultant will have taken them into account before deciding against surgery.

If surgery may become necessary in the future, you should try to stop smoking now, or at least cut right down. Some surgeons will only perform *life-saving* operations on heavy smokers.

However, your hernia may never worsen to the point where an operation becomes necessary. So, in the circumstances, it may well be better to 'wait and see'. You could discuss some self-help measures with your GP as these may help to relieve your symptoms.

Any operation has a certain risk – however small – and you should consider the alternative forms of treatment first. If you still feel you want your hernia repaired surgically, you could ask your doctor if you can see another consultant. Your age and smoking habits would probably preclude the use of a general anaesthetic for any operation, but an alternative may be feasible.

6.   I have waited over a year for my hernia operation, and have still not been given a date for it. The last date had to be cancelled. Can I do anything to speed things up?

Even if you are learning to live with your hernia, waiting like this can be stressful. Do write to the consultant whose list you are on. It may be possible to put you on a standby list, or at least to give you some idea of how long you may have to wait.

If you do not get a satisfactory response from your consultant, you could ask your GP if another consultant in your area has a shorter waiting list. If you are still not satisfied, your local Community Health Council may be able to advise you. Your local hospital or Citizens Advice Bureau will have their address.

7. *I am due to have a hernia operation next month as a day-case patient. Since seeing the consultant, my circumstances have changed and there will be no one to look after me when I come home from hospital. Shall I just go as a day case anyway and hope that I can manage?*

You should contact your doctor or the consultant's secretary to explain your altered situation. You would probably not be allowed to go home after day-case surgery without a competent adult to care for you, so it is better to discuss this now. You may have to stay in hospital overnight after your operation, and another date may have to be fixed for it.

8. *The waiting list for hernia operations is over a year at my local hospital. Can I ask to be treated at another hospital with a shorter waiting list in the same or another area?*

Although you can be treated at another hospital in your area, you should talk to your GP about this. Your doctor may feel that the consultant chosen to treat you is the best for your particular operation. If your hernia is not very troublesome, it may be worth waiting.

In theory, you can ask to be treated at a hospital outside your health region. In practice, however, this is now almost impossible. The administrators of the recently set-up independent hospital trusts are not keen to pay for services in other districts.

9. I have health insurance which covers consultants' fees and hospitalisation costs for a hernia operation. Will there be any other costs I will have to pay myself?

Your insurance should cover all your hospital costs, including any tests you have to have, medicines and meals while you are in hospital. The bill will be sent directly to your insurance company. Before leaving the hospital, you will have to pay yourself for any extra food you have had (e.g. for visitors), for any alcohol such as wine with your meals, for personal laundry other than sheets and hospital gowns, for postage, and for any telephone calls you have made.

It is a good idea to ask the hospital for a written list of charges for which you would be liable. If you are in any doubt about what your insurance covers, check with your insurance company and ask for details in writing. Some types of policy exclude certain costs. You could also ask staff at the hospital to check your policy for you.

It is also worth finding out who pays if any complications arise and you have to stay in hospital longer than anticipated. Most insurance policies will cover further treatment necessary as a direct result of your operation, or further complications related to it, but will not pay for anything which arises while you are in hospital but which is not connected directly with your original condition.

10. I am a teacher, and would like to have my operation during the school holidays. Would this be possible?

Ask your doctor to mention this in the letter to the consultant. Most hospitals will try to fit your operation in at a convenient time, although it is not always possible.

11. I have been told that it will be at least 9 months before I can have my operation. I am keen to have it sooner, and would be prepared to pay myself. How long would I have to wait if I went to a private hospital?

Once you have seen your GP, it should take no more than a week to arrange an appointment with a private consultant. You should be able to be admitted to a private hospital a week or two later, or any time after this that suits you.

12. I am due to enter hospital for a hernia operation as a day case. Will my doctor visit me at home as a matter of routine?

In some areas, a district nurse or GP may call to see patients who have had operations as day cases, but it is more likely that this will not happen, and, indeed, it is not normally necessary.

If you are worried at all, and are unable to get to your doctor's surgery, ring and ask if a home visit can be arranged for you.

13. How long will I be in hospital?

Unless you are being treated as a day case, you will probably be admitted on the day of your operation, and be discharged the following day. Elderly people may be asked to enter hospital on the day before their operation so that any necessary tests and investigations can be carried out, and the results received before surgery. This is to exclude the possibility of any heart or chest complaint (more common in this age group) that would make the use of a general anaesthetic inadvisable.

14. I do not want to have a general anaesthetic for my operation. Is there an alternative?

If you have not already seen a consultant at an out-patient clinic, mention this when you do. Otherwise, tell the anaesthetist who will see you in hospital before your operation. You could also tell the nurse who admits you to the hospital ward, as she will be able to ask the anaesthetist to visit you to discuss this.

There are alternatives to general anaesthesia, such as a spinal injection or other forms of local anaesthetic. You would probably be given a sedative as well, to relax you and/or put you into a light sleep during surgery. The anaesthetist will be able to discuss the possibilities with you, and should certainly view your preference sympathetically.

15. When will I be able to return to work after my operation?

The recovery period varies from person to person. Your GP should be able to give you a rough idea beforehand. If your work does not include lifting or carrying heavy objects, you should be able to return to work after a couple of weeks at most. Heavy manual labourers may need 6 to 8 weeks off work to make sure they do not re-open their wounds before they have healed properly.

16. Should I stay in bed for a few days after my operation?

It is important that you move around and walk a little as soon as possible after surgery. This reduces the chances of a blood clot developing in a vein. Although blood clots normally dissolve of their own accord, they can become detached from the wall of the vein and find their way to the heart or lungs. If this does happen, they can be fatal. Exercise helps to keep the blood flowing through the veins and to prevent clots forming.

So, although you will find you need to rest after your operation, it is better to get up at regular intervals and walk about. Staying in bed is not a good idea – and should not be necessary.

17. Will my wound be very painful?

Some people find they do not need to take any painkillers after their first or second post-operative day. Others continue to need them for several days. It is not really clear why this varies; but tablets such as aspirin or paracetamol should be sufficient to control any pain or discomfort if taken regularly. If you have severe pain after the first couple of days, contact your GP to make sure that no complication has arisen.

18. Will it be all right for me to drive myself home after my operation?

Even if you are discharged from hospital on the day after your operation and feel all right, you are *not* safe to drive. You would be unable to stop quickly in an emergency and, if you have had a general anaesthetic, its effects can last for several days. Your insurance will probably be invalid for at least 48 hours after surgery.

You may be advised to wait a couple of weeks before driving, but should at least wait until you would be able to use the brake in an emergency without being affected by pain or stiffness in your wound.

19. Can I have a bath after my operation?

If your wound has been covered with an adhesive strip of transparent dressing, you will be able to shower before the stitches are removed. You should not have a bath during this time as the wound should not be soaked until it has healed.

With any other type of dressing, you should not bath or shower until your stitches have been removed or your wound has been seen by your doctor – about 10 days after your operation.

20. I had my operation 3 days ago. A painful, large swelling has now come up near the wound. What should I do?

This may be a haematoma – a blood-filled swelling possibly caused by damage to a blood vessel during the operation. Although it is best to contact your GP to check this, it is unlikely to cause any further problems and will probably be re-absorbed without the need for treatment.

However, if you develop a temperature or pain and inflammation, your wound may have become infected and you should seek medical attention.

21. I have recently had an emergency operation for a strangulated hernia. My wound has swollen and become red and sore, and I have a temperature. Should I tell my doctor?

You should contact your doctor or consultant surgeon immediately. Your wound may have become infected and, if so, will require treatment.

22. I had a hernia operation a week ago, but still have numbness and 'pins and needles' around the operation site. Is this normal?

Numbness of this sort can last for several months, and is likely to be due to minor nerve damage during the operation. However, if it continues and the site of your wound becomes painful, you should ask you doctor to have a look at it. Neuromas caused by regrowing damaged nerves are rare, but if a neuroma does develop, it may need to be removed surgically. Always make an appointment to see your GP if you are worried.

23. Since coming home after my operation, quite severe bruising has developed around the wound, the appearance of which is quite shocking. What has caused this and what should I do about it?

Although bruising can be distressing when it is extensive, it is usually a relatively minor post-operative complication. It often does not appear immediately, and is due to bleeding (haemorrhage) under the skin. It is common following operations in which small blood vessels have been cut. It may last for several days. However, if the bruising continues to get worse, or if you are concerned about it, contact your doctor for advice.

Case histories

The case histories which follow are not intended to make any specific point. They have been chosen at random as examples of the different experiences of four different people. They are included simply to illustrate the reality of having a hernia for these people, and how their experiences of similar operations varied.

CASE 1

Norman was 64 when he had a hernia repair operation, and was working as a caretaker and porter. He had suffered from a slight ache in his groin for many years, but it was not until a lump developed that he decided to visit his GP. The lump would appear while he was working, but disappear again as soon as he rested.

His GP said an operation would be necessary, but that Norman could continue to work for the time being. However, Norman was forced to stop work a month later because of severe pain. His doctor advised him to rest as much as possible.

When Norman saw the consultant at his local hospital, the lump was no longer visible, but it was agreed that an operation would be advisable otherwise the hernia was likely to recur as soon as he went back to work.

Within a month, Norman was admitted to hospital on the day before his operation so that some routine tests could be carried out which were necessary because of his age. These revealed a slight heart murmur, and it was decided that a spinal anaesthetic would be safer than a general one.

On the morning of his operation, Norman was given a pre-med. which made him relaxed and drowsy. A couple of hours later he was wheeled to the operating theatre. He lay on his side while the anaesthetist put a mask over his nose and mouth to deliver a pain-killing gas mixture, and then injected the local anaesthetic into his lower spine. The injection was painless and Norman was soon asleep.

He woke up in the theatre just before he was taken to the recovery room. From there he was returned to his ward. He was numb from the waist down, but felt quite well and pain free. The numbness lasted some 5 to 6 hours, but when it wore off, he still had no more than slight discomfort. He did not require painkillers, either while in hospital or during his recovery at home.

The following day he was discharged home to the care of his wife.

Seven days after his operation, the nurse at Norman's doctor's surgery removed the wound covering and stitches. His wound had healed well. Apart from some minor bruising in his groin, which lasted for several days, he felt only occasional, slight discomfort; some numbness remained in his groin 10 days after surgery.

Norman's doctor advised him to remain away from work for at least another 6 weeks due to the heavy lifting and carrying involved in his job.

Norman admits to having been fearful of the anaesthetic as he had never had one before, and he was happy to have been given a spinal rather than a general one. He feels that the operation was well worthwhile; he had no post-operative problems, and made a steady recovery.

CASE 2

Susan is 49, and the mother of two adult children. She is self-employed, teaching computer training courses.

Some 6 months before Susan's operation to repair an umbilical hernia, she noticed a small, grape-sized lump on her navel. The lump could be pushed flat, but soon protruded again and became painful when she was tired.

Susan went to her GP, who arranged for her to see a consultant, although he did stress that there was no urgent need for treatment. When she saw the consultant a couple of months later, he suggested that Susan should have an operation to repair the hernia as it was likely to increase in size and become more painful with time. He explained to her what the operation would involve.

About 2 months later, the hospital sent Susan a date for her operation, but as this was inconvenient for her due to her workload at that time, they agreed to alter it. Another appointment was made a few weeks later. However, 2 days before Susan was due to enter hospital, she was telephoned and told that her operation had had to be cancelled and another appointment would be made for her as soon as possible. A month later Susan telephoned her consultant's secretary and was fitted into a gap in the operating list within a few days.

During the weeks before her operation, Susan soon learnt which activities caused her hernia to become painful, and tried to avoid them. Unfortunately, her work involves a good deal of standing, and this was one of the main, unavoidable, causes of pain for her. She also found that lifting heavy objects, such as joints of meat etc. in and out of the oven, put a strain on her abdomen and made the hernia protrude.

At her out-patients' appointment the consultant had raised the possibility of Susan's operation being done as a day case, and this had led her to believe that the operation itself and the period of recovery from it would all be over within a few days. She was surprised, and somewhat distressed, to learn from her GP that she might have to be off work for up to 3 months after surgery. As her job sometimes involves driving long distances, she was warned that she might not be fit to do this for several weeks after her operation.

Day-case surgery turned out to be unsuitable for Susan as she had previously had an allergic reaction to a commonly used anaesthetic. Because of this, she was asked to go into hospital the day before her operation was to take place so that the anaesthetist could discuss her medical history and anaesthesia with her. The operation during which her allergy had been discovered some years earlier had been done at the same hospital, and by the time Susan was admitted for her hernia repair, the anaesthetist had read the notes concerning her allergic reaction. He was therefore able to discuss this with Susan, and reassure her about the general anaesthetic she would be given.

Before entering hospital, Susan had expected to be home again the day after her operation, but when she was admitted she was told this would be unlikely, as her bladder and bowel, which would probably be moved during surgery, would have to be working properly again before she could be discharged.

As Susan had previously suffered a blood clot, she was given anti-embolism stockings as soon as she was admitted to the hospital ward, and had to wear these until she left hospital 5 days later.

The operation was done the day after she was admitted, and Susan spent the rest of that day dozing and sleeping. When she left the recovery room, she was given oxygen through a mask to help her to breathe. She continued to use this for a few hours. Susan did not feel sick when she came round from the anaesthetic, and was able to eat breakfast as normal the next morning.

During the night following her operation, Susan awoke with

an urgent need to urinate, but was unable to do so. Early the next morning, a bladder catheter was inserted – a slightly uncomfortable but quickly completed procedure – and the nurses on her ward kept a careful watch on the amount of urine she produced through the catheter.

That night, the catheter was removed, and the next morning Susan was able to urinate unaided. This was also the first day that she was able to get out of bed.

The day after her operation, Susan developed a temperature, and a fan was placed by her bed to try to cool her down. By the evening, her temperature had begun to fall. The next day, her blood pressure rose suddenly, and the day after that her temperature increased again. As it had begun to fall by the next day when the doctor saw her, she was able to go home.

Susan did admit to feeling rather 'abandoned' and anxious when she left hospital as she had little information about what to expect during her recovery period.

Although she was given painkillers regularly while she was in hospital, she only needed them in the mornings and before she went to sleep at night for the first week she was at home.

When Susan had been at home for a couple of days, a large red lump appeared at each end of her wound where the looped ends of the stitches emerged from under the skin. There was also a red patch of inflammation on her stomach near the wound. Susan's temperature and blood pressure continued to rise and fall. A week after her operation, she visited her GP who gave her antibiotics to control the inflammation and swelling.

The subcutaneous stitches were removed by the GP practice nurse 2 weeks after Susan's operation, and her wound had healed well.

A week later, Susan was feeling quite well, although she became easily tired. She found, for example, that she could do the vacuuming without too much discomfort, but it still made her wound ache, and left her feeling weary.

She planned to attempt short journeys driving her car about 4 weeks after her operation. Before that time, she had not felt confident that she would be able to do an emergency stop if required. Longer trips, she thought, would probably have to wait a little longer, until she became less easily tired.

After her operation, Susan visited her GP every 2 weeks to get the certificates she needed to claim sickness benefit. She took each day as it came, waiting as patiently as she could until she felt fit to do her work properly again.

CASE 3

At the time of his operation, David was 38 years old; a healthy, active man and a keen rugby player. About 3 years earlier he had noticed an ache and a small, soft swelling in his right groin above the skinfold. The ache gradually became worse over the next couple of years, and, suspecting he had a hernia, David visited his GP, who thought it was better left untreated at that stage.

However, the lump grew larger and harder, and the hernia became more difficult to push back through the muscle wall. Concerned about the danger of a strangulated hernia, David again went to see his GP, who arranged for him to see a consultant. His hernia was now more painful and had begun to affect his lifestyle; he was careful to avoid any activity which would make it hurt, such as playing rugby.

A couple of weeks later, he saw a surgeon at his local hospital who agreed that the hernia should be repaired. As David was otherwise fit, it was suggested that the operation be done as a day case. A urine sample was taken and his blood pressure was checked at this out-patients' appointment.

A few weeks later, David was admitted to a ward in his local hospital at 8 a.m. The surgeon visited him there and explained what his operation would entail. Having shaved his groin and put on his hospital gown and anti-embolism stockings, he was wheeled to the anaesthetic room. By 10 a.m., he had been given a general anaesthetic and was ready for the operation.

Less than an hour later, he woke up in the recovery room, where he was visited by the consultant surgeon who warned him that his groin would be tender the next day. David was then returned to the ward, where he was seen by the surgeon who had performed the operation.

Once he had passed urine, he was able to be collected by his wife later that afternoon. As he was still feeling groggy and his wound was quite painful, his wife asked the nursing staff for a wheelchair to transport him to the hospital exit.

Before leaving the hospital, David asked a nurse whether he should take laxatives to avoid putting any strain on his wound for the next couple of days. He was given 2 days' supply of painkillers, and told to contact his GP if he felt he needed a laxative.

Later that evening, the local anaesthetic which had been injected into his wound during the operation began to wear off, and, despite taking regular pain-killing tablets, the tenderness in his groin persisted.

David and his wife had assumed that they would be visited at home by a district nurse or doctor, and were dismayed to discover that, as in most areas, this is not the case unless such a visit has been previously arranged.

The next day, the area around the wound was swollen and numb. One side of David's penis and scrotum felt very tender and the skin was pink. The consultant surgeon later explained that the sensation of bruising was due to pressure on the soft tissues during surgery. The pink coloration of the skin was caused by a dye in the sterile antiseptic agent used pre-operatively, and could be washed off with soap and water.

For several days after his operation, the discomfort and

tenderness continued, and were partcularly troublesome at night when he was trying to settle in bed.

The swelling gradually became a large, hard lump; a vein in David's inner thigh also swelled, and the area of numbness spread. After a couple of days, while his wife was at work, he rang his GP to ask for a home visit. When his GP did visit him later that day, she arranged for an ambulance to take him back to hospital for a check-up.

The surgeon who had performed the operation examined David, but decided the swelling was nothing to worry about; he reassured him and sent him home.

Although the lump increased in size for a day or two, and continued to be tender and painful, it had begun to shrink by the time David saw the consultant at the out-patients' clinic a week after his operation. By this time, he had removed the wound covering himself, and the wound could be seen to be healing well.

Two weeks after his operation, David was able to return to his office work. He could walk quite comfortably, but found standing for any length of time caused aching and a slight hard swelling in his groin. He still had 'pins and needles' on his inner thigh, but the area in which this occurred was gradually decreasing.

David found the unexpected swelling and numbness worrying, and was frustrated by the difficulty he experienced in simple manouevres such as getting into and out of bed in the first few days after his operation.

CASE 4

Marion had her operation at the age of 82. She is married and has two sons.

About 4 years before her operation, Marion's husband had collapsed beside the toilet, and Marion had to pull him up.

Soon afterwards she noticed a small, soft swelling in her groin which disappeared when she lay flat. It gradually grew larger and harder, and ached when she was tired or stood for a long time. She mentioned it to her doctor, who decided it was best left alone. He warned her, however, that if the hernia began to be painful or could no longer be pushed back, she should contact him at once.

About 3 years after the swelling first appeared, a consultant who was examining Marion for another medical problem noticed her hernia, now the size of a tennis ball. He suggested it should be repaired to avoid the risk of complications such as strangulation of the bowel.

Marion was put on a waiting list and entered hospital a few months later on the day before her operation was scheduled. During that day, she underwent some routine tests – blood and urine tests, electrocardiography, and blood pressure measurement. The following morning, as she got ready to go to the operating theatre, a doctor came to the ward to tell her that her operation had had to be cancelled as her blood test had revealed a very low iron content.

She was put on a course of iron tablets, and recalled to hospital a few months later. Again, she was admitted the day before her operation, and all the tests were repeated. The next morning, her false teeth were removed and she was given a pre-med. before being taken to the operating theatre.

She slept for most of the day after the operation, and awoke during the night feeling slightly nauseated, but with no more than minor discomfort from her wound. She was given pain-killing tablets while in hospital, where she remained for a further 2 days. During this time she was given a built-up toilet seat to use as she found lowering herself down to sit on the toilet caused pain in her wound.

Once Marion was at home, she did not need any further painkillers, and found the wound caused her very little discomfort.

The district nurse came to her house 10 days after the operation to remove the stitches. The nurse put an adhesive strip over the wound as a small part of it was not completely healed. She told Marion not to have a bath until healing was complete.

Marion is pleased to have had her hernia repaired and feels that her operation and recovery went well. She had been anxious for some time about the possibility of complications arising and of having to be taken to hospital for emergency surgery without first being able to make arrangements for someone to care for her husband.

Medical terms

Abdomen/Abdominal cavity The body cavity between the diaphragm and the floor of the pelvis which contains the digestive organs – the stomach and intestines.

Abdominal Associated with the abdomen.

Absorbable stitches Stitches which are made of a material which is able to dissolve in the tissues, such as catgut and Vicryl. Absorbable stitches do not, therefore, need to be removed.

Acid reflux The backwards flow of acid produced in the stomach. Acid passes back up the oesophagus towards the mouth, causing the discomfort of heartburn.

Acquired A term used to describe a condition which was not present at birth, but which developed afterwards.

Allergy An over-sensitivity to a particular substance which causes the body to react against it. The allergic reaction may be mild, such as an itchy rash, or it may be more severe, involving fainting, vomiting or loss of consciousness. Your doctor should be told about any allergies you have so that they can be added to your medical records.

Anaesthetic A drug used to cause loss of sensation or feeling in part of the body.

Analgesic A drug which blocks sensations of pain; a painkiller.

Anatomy The structure of living organisms; the study of body structure.

Antacid A substance which reduces or neutralises acidity. Antacids are used to neutralise the acid secreted by the stomach and thus to relieve the symptoms of indigestion and heartburn caused by this acid as it flows back into the oesophagus.

Ante-natal screening   Tests carried out before the birth of a baby to detect any abnormalities.

Antibiotic   A substance which kills germs. Antibiotics were originally extracted from various bacteria and fungi, but many are now produced synthetically.

Anticoagulant   A substance which prevents blood from clotting (coagulating), for example heparin. Heparin is given by subcutaneous injection to patients who are at a high risk of developing deep vein thrombosis during their stay in hospital.

Anti-embolism stockings/Thrombo-embolic deterrent stockings (TEDS)   Stockings worn by a patient throughout an operation to help prevent blood clots forming in the deep veins of the legs by assisting the circulation of blood within them.

Anti-emetic   A drug which helps to stop you feeling sick.

Appendicectomy   Surgical removal of the appendix.

Bile   A greenish yellow fluid secreted by the liver which helps to keep the contents of the intestines alkaline and to digest fat.

Bowel   Another name for the gut.

Bruise   The discoloration caused by blood accumulating in the tissues under the skin in the area of an injury.

Cannula   A very fine tube or needle which is inserted into a vein, usually in the back of the hand. Cannulas are used to introduce or remove fluids from the body, and to administer drugs such as anaesthetics. They are usually made of plastic, but can be glass or metal.

Catheter   A tube for withdrawing or introducing fluid into a body cavity.

Cautery/Cauterisation See **Electrocautery**.

Colon   The first and largest part of the large intestine between its junctions with the small intestine and with the rectum.

Complication   A condition which occurs as the result of another disease or condition. A complication may also be an unwanted side-effect of treatment.

Congenital Something that has been present since before, or from the time of, birth; inherited.

Consent form A form which patients must sign before surgery to confirm that their treatment has been explained to them, and that they have given their permission for the operation and anaesthesia.

Constipation A condition in which opening of the bowels is difficult and infrequent.

Contraceptive pill A drug taken orally to prevent conception taking place.

Coronary thrombosis A blood clot within an artery of the heart which may be the cause of a heart attack.

Cosmetic scar A scar which is not easily apparent and which is achieved, for example, by stitching the wound subcutaneously, i.e. under the surface of the skin.

Crepitus The sound made when two rough surfaces rub against each other, or when pressure is put on tissues filled with gas or air. Gas which has been introduced into the abdominal cavity during laparoscopic hernia repair can escape into the area around the hernia, causing swelling in the groin. This swelling has the characteristic 'crackling' feel of crepitus.

Day-case surgery A minor operation carried out on a patient who is in hospital for one day only, with no overnight stay.

Deep vein thrombosis A blood clot in the deep veins of the leg.

Defect A deficiency; used in the context of this book to mean a hole in the muscle wall.

Depilatory cream Hair-removing cream sometimes used as an alternative to shaving.

Diagnosis The identification of a disease based on its symptoms and signs.

Diaphragm A layer of tissue, particularly muscle, stretched across an opening. This term is normally used for the muscular sheet which separates the thoracic and abdominal cavities and assists in breathing.

Diaphragmatic hernia   A rare type of hernia which occurs in the upper abdomen.

Diathermy   The process by which heat is applied to the tissues during an operation to stop bleeding. The heat is usually provided by a high-frequency electrical current. Diathermy is used to seal the ends of blood vessels during an operation.

Digestive organs   The organs involved in breaking down food into small units which can be absorbed. The main digestive organs are the stomach, intestines, liver and pancreas.

Discharge letter   The letter given to patients as they leave hospital. This letter gives details of their treatment and any other information of which their family doctor should be aware.

Dissection   The separation or division of tissues or organs during a surgical operation.

Dissolvable stitches   See **Absorbable stitches**.

Distension   Enlargement or dilatation.

Divarication of the recti   Separation or stretching of the vertical rectus muscles in the abdomen.

Duodenum   The first part of the small intestine, which is about 20–25 cm (8–10 inches) long. The duodenum begins at the end of the stomach.

Dysphagia   Difficulty in swallowing.

Eczema   Inflammation of the skin causing itching and burning.

Eczematous   Resembling or connected with eczema.

Electrocardiogram (ECG)   A record of the activity of the heart as a series of electrical wave patterns produced prior to the muscles in the heart shortening (contracting).

Electrocardiography   The process by which an electrocardiogram is recorded. Electrodes are taped to the skin over the heart and detect the electrical activity of the heart muscle.

Electrocautery/Cautery/Cauterisation   The process used to control bleeding during an operation. An electrical current heats the end of an instrument which, when applied to the tiny blood vessels, seals them and stops them bleeding.

Embolism   The sudden blocking of a blood vessel by a blood clot or air bubble.

Embolus (plural: **emboli**)   A blood clot, or an air bubble, which blocks a blood vessel.

Endoscope   An instrument for viewing hollow organs which can be inserted inside the organs themselves.

Endoscopy   The examination of hollow organs using an endoscope.

Epidural anaesthetic   A local anaesthetic which is injected into the space around the spinal cord and numbs the back, lower abdomen and legs.

Epigastric hernia   A hernia which protrudes through the central abdominal muscle between the navel and the breastbone. Epigastric hernias are usually filled with fat.

Excision   Removal of a part by cutting it out or away.

Exomphalos   A type of large umbilical hernia recognised at birth in which the intestine protrudes through the umbilicus.

Expire   To breathe out.

Femoral canal   A canal which runs alongside the thigh bone (femur) in the leg adjacent to the femoral vein.

Femoral hernia   A hernia into the femoral canal in the lower groin.

Fetus   A developing embryo.

Fever   The reaction of the body to infection, which includes raised body temperature, a flushed skin, and increased pulse and breathing rates.

Field block   Injection of an anaesthetic around the site of an operation. Nerves follow a predictable path, and can be blocked in specific areas, or 'fields', near the operation site.

Fundus   The part of a hernia which is farthest away from its neck.

Gangrene   The death and decomposition of tissue caused when its blood supply has been cut off.

Gastrointestinal tract   The stomach and intestines; the gut.

General anaesthetic A drug which puts you to sleep so that you have no sensation in any part of your body.

Groin The groove between the lower part of the abdomen and the thigh.

Gullet See **Oesophagus**.

Gut See **Gastrointestinal tract**.

Haematoma A blood-filled swelling. Haematomas can form after surgery if a blood vessel continues to bleed. When the blood is spread in the tissues it appears as a bruise.

Haemophilia An inherited disorder of the blood-clotting mechanism of the body which prevents the blood from clotting naturally. Haemophilia is transmitted by women, but normally only affects men.

Haemorrhage Bleeding; the escape of blood from arteries or veins in any part of the body.

Heartburn A burning feeling in the throat caused by regurgitation of the stomach contents.

Hernia The bulging of one (or more) of the body's internal organs through a weakness in the muscle wall of the body cavity.

Herniate To push through a cavity wall; to form a hernia.

Herniography A test to detect the presence of a hernia. A dye is injected into the abdominal cavity which will fill the hernial sac, if present. The dye can be seen on X-ray, and thus the hernia is highlighted.

Hernioplasty The operation to return the contents of a hernia to their natural position.

Herniorrhaphy The process by which a hernia is repaired. The protruding tissue is replaced, and the muscle wall is sewn and strengthened.

Herniotomy The operation to reduce a hernia by opening and excising its sac.

Hiatus An opening.

Hiatus hernia A hernia involving the protrusion of part of the stomach through an opening in the diaphragm.

Hormone replacement therapy (HRT) Treatment which attempts to correct an imbalance in the hormones present in the body, such as occurs in women at the menopause.

Ileum The lower part of the small intestine which runs from the jejunum to the colon.

Impacted Firmly wedged.

Incision A cut or wound made by a sharp instrument, such as during an operation.

Incisional hernia A hernia which occurs through a weakness in the muscle wall caused by previous surgery.

Indigestion Discomfort or pain caused by disturbance of the normal digestion of food.

Induction agent A drug which brings on sleep.

Inflammation Increase in blood flow causing redness, heat, pain and swelling of a tissue in response to injury or infection.

Inguinal canal The canal through which the testicles descend to the scrotum. The canal passes through the groin (inguinal = relating to the groin).

Inguinal hernia A hernia in the groin in the area of the inguinal canal. Inguinal hernias can be direct or indirect.

Inhalational anaesthetic A drug in the form of a gas which is breathed in through a face mask.

Intravenous Introduced into the body by injection into a vein.

Irreducible hernia A hernia which cannot be pushed back through a hole in the muscle wall.

'Keyhole surgery' A colloquial name for minimally invasive or laparoscopic surgery.

Laparoscope A telescope-like instrument with a light source and a camera attached which can be introduced into the abdominal cavity. It allows examination of the peritoneum and internal organs without the need for a large incision to be made in the body.

Laparoscopic surgery Surgery carried out with the aid of a laparoscope. It involves making a series of small incisions in the body wall through which the laparoscope and surgical instruments can be inserted. A video camera and a light source are introduced with the laparoscope, which enable the surgeon to see the inside of the body on a video screen.

Laparoscopy   The examination of the abdominal cavity using a laparoscope, which is inserted through a small incision made in the abdominal wall.

Laparotomy   The operation to explore the peritoneal cavity, for example to look for evidence of a hernia following signs of obstruction or strangulation of the bowel. Laparotomy involves making a long incision in the abdominal wall so that the surgeon can examine the abdominal cavity.

Laxative   A drug which aids the evacuation of faeces. Laxatives are useful in the short-term relief of constipation.

Local anaesthetic   A drug which blocks the sensation in the area around which it is injected, causing numbness.

Maintenance agent   A drug which keeps you asleep.

Medical history   Details of someone's past health, including illnesses, operations, allergies etc.

Medical treatment   Treatment which does not involve surgery.

Monitoring equipment   Equipment used to watch over (monitor) the various activities of the body, such as the heart beat, breathing rate etc.

Minimally invasive surgery   Another name for laparoscopic surgery (see above), which involves a much less invasive technique than conventional surgery.

'Named nurse'   A nurse allocated to a particular patient who is responsible for that patient's nursing throughout their stay in hospital. 'Named nurses' were introduced under the terms of the Government's Patients' Charter.

Nausea   A feeling of sickness.

Navel   The umbilicus; the dip in the surface of the abdomen where the umbilical cord was attached to the fetus.

Necrosis   Death of part of a tissue.

Neuroma A swelling which may cause pain and is due to regrowing nerve fibres following injury to a nerve.

Nil by mouth A term used to mean that nothing – neither food nor drink – must be swallowed in the hours before an operation.

Non-absorbable stitches Stitches made of a material which will not dissolve. These stitches need to be removed once the wound has healed or, if they are used internally, remain in place forever.

Non-traumatic hernia A hernia which is caused by something other than injury.

Obesity An excessive amount of fat in the body. Obesity is usually measured on height and weight tables.

Obstructed hernia A hernia which has become squeezed through a small hole in the muscle wall. When the hernia contains part of the intestine, obstruction cuts off the passage of the intestinal contents, causing a blockage.

Oesophageal sphincter A valve at the end of the oesophagus where it joins the stomach. It prevents the passage of food back towards the mouth.

Oesophagus The gullet; the tube which carries food from the back of the mouth to the opening at the top of the stomach.

Oesophagitis Inflammation of the oesophagus, often caused by reflux of the stomach contents – **reflux oesophagitis**.

Organ A group of cells which are organised to form part of the body with a specific function, e.g. the heart or stomach.

Osteitis Inflammation of a bone.

Para-umbilical hernia A hernia through the abdominal wall above or below the navel.

Pelvis/Pelvic cavity The cavity between the lower abdomen and groin which contains the bladder, lower rectum and some reproductive organs. (The pelvis is also the name given to the basin-shaped ring of bone which forms the hips.)

Peritoneum The membrane which lines the abdominal cavity and the upper pelvic cavity. It also forms a layer over the organs within these cavities.

Peritonitis   Inflammation of the peritoneum caused by bacterial infection.

Port   A narrow tube which is inserted through a small hole in the body wall, for example in the abdomen during laparoscopic hernia repair. A valve is attached to this tube which allows gas and surgical instruments to be introduced into and removed from the body cavity without the loss of the gas used to inflate it.

Post-operative   After an operation.

Predisposing factor   Something which makes one susceptible to a particular disease or condition.

'Pre-med.'/Pre-medication   Any drug which is given before another, e.g. a drug given before an anaesthetic to reduce the patient's anxiety by making them relaxed and drowsy.

Pre-operative   Before an operation.

Prostate gland   A gland which surrounds the neck of the bladder in men, and which secretes a sperm-activating fluid. The prostate gland often becomes enlarged in elderly men, causing constriction of the neck of the bladder and thus retention of urine, particularly after hernia repair.

Pulse oximeter   A device which measures the amount of oxygen in the blood.

Recovery room   A ward near the operating theatre where patients are taken to recover from the anaesthetic after surgery. The recovery room is staffed by nurses who are specially trained in this type of care.

Rectum   The last part of the large intestine between the colon and anus.

Rectus (plural: **recti**)   The abdominal rectus muscle is a vertical column of flat muscle in the abdomen. There is a strap of rectus muscle on either side of the midline.

Recurrence   The reappearance of symptoms after a period of absence, for example after hernia repair.

Reducible hernia   A hernia whose contents can be pushed back into their correct position.

Reduction Restoration of organs or tissues to their correct position.

Reflux Flow in a backwards direction; regurgitation.

Regurgitation The process by which food which has already been swallowed returns from the stomach towards the mouth.

Resection The cutting out of part of an organ or tissue.

Rheumatoid arthritis Inflammation of the joints, the specific cause of which is unknown.

Richter's hernia Protrusion of a small piece of the intestinal wall into a hernial sac with strangulation. Most of the circumference of the gut remains in place in the abdomen, and therefore obstruction does not occur.

Rolling hiatus hernia A relatively uncommon type of hiatus hernia which causes flatulence, and possibly difficulty in swallowing.

Scrotum The pouch of skin below the penis which contains the testes.

Sedative A drug which slows down the activity of a part or the whole of the body.

Seminal vesicle The tube which carries sperm from the testicle to the vas deferens.

Side-effect An unwanted effect that accompanies another disease or treatment.

Sign Something a doctor looks for as evidence of disease or medical abnormality, for example swelling or bleeding.

Sliding hiatus hernia The most common type of hiatus hernia which involves regurgitation of acid from the stomach into the gullet, causing heartburn.

Spermatic cord The cord in the scrotum which carries sperm from the testicle, together with arteries and veins.

Spinal anaesthetic A drug which is injected between the bones of the spine into the space around the nerves, and which causes numbness in the legs, lower abdomen and bottom.

Step-down ward A ward to which day-case patients go in some hospitals to recover before going home after an operation.

Sternum   The breastbone.

Strangulated hernia   A hernia in which the blood supply has become constricted, which may lead to gangrene and perforation of the hernia's contents.

Stricture   Narrowing of a passage.

Subcutaneous   Under the surface of the skin.

Subcuticular stitches   Stitches which are made under the skin in order to give a less noticeable, cosmetic scar.

Surgical treatment   Treatment of disease or injury by means of an operation.

Suture   A surgical stitch or row of stitches.

Symptom   A disturbance to the normal working of the body which is not necessarily visible but is felt by the patient, such as pain or tiredness.

Testicle   The organ in which sperm develop; the testis.

Thorax/Thoracic cavity   The cavity between the neck and the abdomen; the chest.

Thrombo-embolic stockings   See **Anti-embolism stockings**

Thrombosis   A blood clot in a vein or artery.

Trachea   The rigid tube which carries air from the mouth towards the lungs; the windpipe.

Truss   A strap-like device worn to control a hernia.

Umbilical hernia   A congenital hernia which occurs in babies. If the muscle wall does not develop fully before birth, part of the contents of the abdomen can protrude through it.

Umbilicus   The navel.

Urethra   The tube through which urine passes as it is discharged from the bladder.

Urine retention   The inability to urinate which can occur following an operation such as that for an inguinal hernia.

Valve   Something which controls the flow of a liquid (or gas) so that it goes in one direction only.

Vas deferens   The tube which carries sperm from the testicle to the penis in men.

How to complain

If you are unhappy about anything that has occurred – or, indeed, that has not occurred – during your stay in hospital, there are several possible paths to follow if you want to make a complaint.

However, before you set the complaints machinery in motion, you should give careful thought to what is involved. Once a formal complaint has been made against a doctor and the complaints procedure has begun, there is little chance of stopping it.

If you think you have a genuine grievance, do try to talk to the person concerned, explaining as clearly and unemotionally as possible what it is that you feel has gone wrong. If you do not feel able to discuss things directly, you can always present your case in a letter.

The vast majority of doctors – GPs and hospital doctors – are dedicated, conscientious and hard working. They really do have their patients' best interests at heart, and many work very long hours each week, night and day. Junior hospital doctors, for example, may have to work up to 100 hours a week, their overtime being compulsory and poorly paid.

A complaint against a doctor is usually a devastating blow, which can cause considerable stress. Of course, if something has gone wrong during your medical treatment, you may also have suffered stress and unhappiness, but before you make an official complaint, do consider whether your doctor's actions have really warranted what many would see as a 'kick in the teeth'.

The best approach is to make a polite and reasoned enquiry to the person concerned. However angry or irritated you may feel, you are likely to find that a complaint made aggressively - however justified this may seem – will be met with a defensive reluctance to co-operate. Medical staff, including GPs, are covered by insurance. If you have ever had a motor accident, you may be familiar with the advice given by insurance companies not to apologise or accept blame, even if you think that the accident was your fault. Medical insurers have the same attitude, which may explain why your normally helpful doctor can appear to be avoiding a simple apology.

Leaflets and other information giving details of all the appropriate councils and complaints procedures and how they work can be obtained from your hospital or local health authority. Your local Citizens' Advice Bureau or Community Health Council will also be able to give you information about what to do and who to go to for help if you have any problems with the offices mentioned here.

HOSPITAL STAFF

If your complaint concerns something that has happened during your stay in hospital, and for some reason you are unable to approach the person directly concerned, you can talk to the ward sister or charge nurse, the hospital doctor on your ward, or the senior manager for the department or ward. Many complaints can be dealt with directly by one of these people, but if this is not possible, they will be able to refer you to the appropriate person.

It is, however, always better to try to sort out any problems by first talking to the person involved, putting your point of view calmly and clearly, and then listening to what they say.

THE GENERAL MANAGER

If you are intimidated by the thought of speaking to one of the people mentioned above, you can write to the hospital's General Manager, sometimes called the Director of Operations or Chief Executive. The General Manager has responsibility for the way the hospital is run.

The Government's Patients' Charter states that anyone making a complaint about an NHS service must receive a 'full and prompt written reply from the Chief Executive or General Manager'. You should therefore receive an immediate response to your letter, and your complaint should be fully investigated by a senior manager.

The hospital switchboard, or any medical or clerical staff at the hospital, should be able to give you the General Manager's name and office address. If you would prefer to do so, you can make an appointment to speak to him or her, rather than writing a letter.

Depending on how serious your complaint is, you should receive either a full report of the investigation into it, or regular letters telling you what is happening until such a report can be made.

Do make sure you keep copies of all letters you write and receive concerning your complaint.

DISTRICT HEALTH AUTHORITY

If the treatment you require is not available in your area, or the waiting list is very long, you can contact your local District Health Authority. The District Health Authority is able to deal with complaints concerning the provision of services, rather than with those resulting from something going wrong with your treatment. The District Health Authority can sometimes arrange for you to have treatment elsewhere where waiting lists are shorter if this is what you want.

Your NHS authority should produce a leaflet to explain how it deals with complaints. This will be available at your hospital or clinic. If you have any difficulty finding out who to contact, write to the general manager of the hospital. The hospital will be able to tell you which health authority covers the area in which you live.

COMMUNITY HEALTH COUNCIL

If you feel that you would like independent advice and assistance, you can obtain this from your local Community Health Council. Someone from the Community Health Council will be able to explain the complaints procedures to you, help you to write letters to the hospital, and also come with you to any meetings arranged between hospital representatives and yourself. Again, the address of the Community Health Council for your area can be obtained from a hospital or local telephone directory.

REGIONAL MEDICAL OFFICER

If your complaint concerns the standard of clinical treatment you received in hospital, and the paths you have already taken have not led to a satisfactory conclusion, you can write to the Regional Medical Officer for your area. The Regional Medical Officer will discuss your complaint with the consultant responsible for your hospital treatment and decide whether a complete review of your case is warranted.

FAMILY HEALTH SERVICES AUTHORITY

Any complaint about a GP which you have been unable to sort out with the doctor in question can be reported to the Family Health Services Authority. Such complaints should be made within 13 weeks of the incident occurring. Again, your local Community Health Council will be able to give you advice, help you make your complaint, and help you to write letters etc.

HEALTH SERVICE COMMISSIONER

If all else has failed, you can take your complaint to the Health Service Commissioner, who deals with complaints made by individuals against the NHS. The Commissioner is independent of both the NHS and the government, being responsible to Parliament.

The Health Service Commissioner is able to deal with complaints concerning the failure of a NHS authority to provide the service it should – a failure which has caused you actual hardship or injustice. However, you must have taken your complaint up with your local health authority first. If you have not received a satisfactory response within a reasonable time, you must enclose copies of all the relevant letters and documents as well as giving details of the incident itself when writing to the Health Service Commissioner. The Health Commissioner is not able to investigate complaints about clinical treatment.

You must also contact the Health Service Commissioner within 1 year of the incident occurring, unless there is some valid reason why you have been unable to do so.

There is a separate Health Service Commissioner for each country within the United Kingdom.

Health Service Commissioner for England
Church House
Great Smith Street
London SW1P 3BW
Telephone: 071–276 2035

Health Service Commissioner for Scotland
Second Floor
11 Melville Crescent
Edinburgh EH3 7LU
Telephone: 031–225 7465

Health Service Commissioner for Wales
4th Floor Pearl Assurance House
Greyfriars Road
Cardiff CF1 3AG
Telephone: 0222–394621

Office of the Northern Ireland Commissioner for Complaints
33 Wellington Place
Belfast BT1 6HN
Telephone: 0232 233821

TAKING LEGAL ACTION

The legal path is likely to be an expensive one, and should be a last resort rather than a starting point.

In theory, everyone has a right to take legal action. However, unless you have very little money and are entitled to Legal Aid, or a great deal of money, you are unlikely to be able to afford this costly process. The outcome of legal action can never be assured, and the possible cost if you lose your case should be borne in mind.

If you do think you have grounds for compensation for injury caused to you as a result of negligence, advice can be sought from:

The Association for the Victims of Medical Accidents (AVMA)
1 London Road
Forest Hill
London SE23 3TP
Telephone: 081 291 2793.

Someone from the AVMA will be able to give you free and confidential legal advice about whether or not you have a case worth pursuing. They will also be able to recommend solicitors with training in medical law who may be prepared to represent you.

Summary

Do tell nursing or other medical staff if you are not happy about *any* aspect of your care in hospital. They may be able to deal with your complaint immediately. But do remember, if your complaint is about a serious matter, or if you are not satisfied with the response you receive, you are entitled to pursue it through all the levels that exist to deal with such problems.

Index